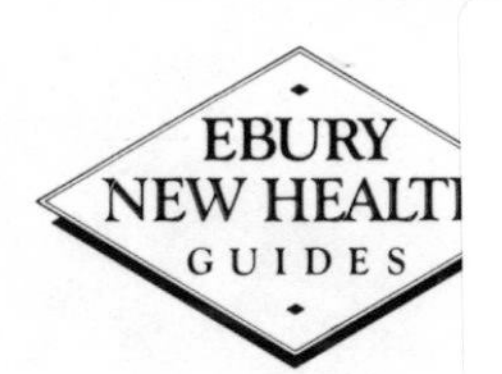
EBURY
NEW HEALT
GUIDES

C000270137

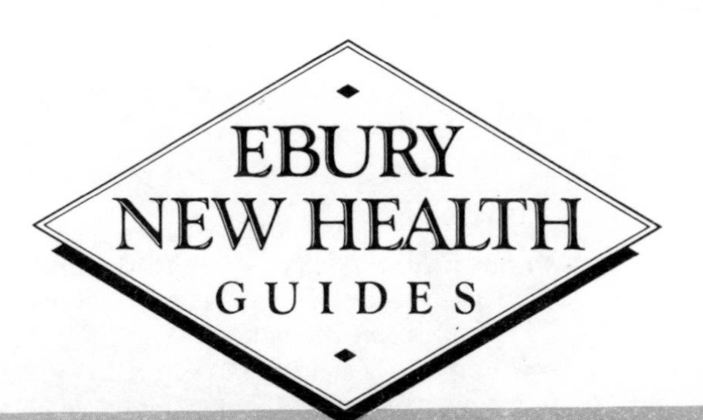

CONQUERING CYSTITIS

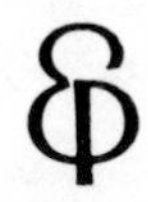

EBURY PRESS LONDON

DR PATRICK KINGSLEY

To LUCY,
who has helped quietly in the background,
yet left me to get on with this book in between
seeing my patients.
To JASON *and* CHRISTOPHER,
whom I hope will make this a better world to
live in.

ACKNOWLEDGEMENTS

The author would like to thank:

Dr. Richard Mackarness who introduced me to a better way of helping patients

Dr. John McLennan, Ontario, Canada, who taught me so much

Mike Franklin who helped me all the time

Phil McCauley who encouraged and enthused me throughout

Hilary Edkins who patiently typed and retyped the manuscript

Published by Ebury Press
Division of the National Magazine Company Ltd
Colquhoun House
27–37 Broadwick Street
London W1V 1FR

ISBN 0 85223 576 3

Edited by Mike Franklin
Designed by Peter Bridgewater Associates
Computerset in Great Britain by
ECM Ltd, London
Printed and bound in Great Britain by
The Bath Press

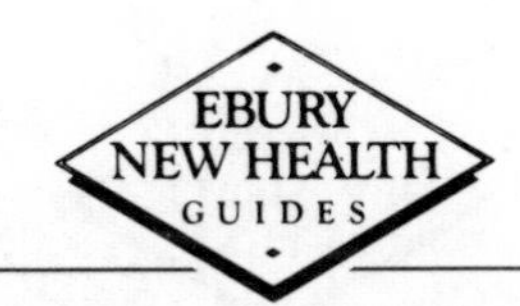

CONTENTS

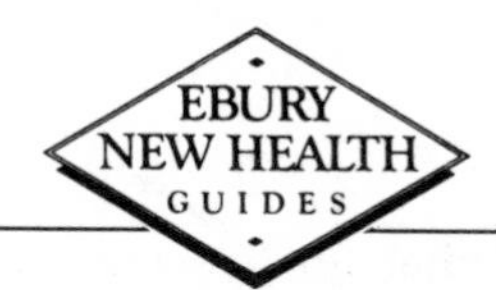

INTRODUCTION

Most people think that cystitis is a simple condition. To someone who has never suffered it, it merely means a slight burning when passing water for which the doctor gives an antibiotic. In fact, frequent episodes of cystitis, known as recurrent or chronic cystitis, can not only be very painful and debilitating but can also affect a sufferer's whole life and make her – most sufferers are women – fear the next attack.

The orthodox view of cystitis is that there is an infection in the patient's bladder and that antibiotics form the backbone of treatment. If frequent attacks occur, the general practitioner will ask the local specialist to see the patient. The treatment will concentrate on the bladder, but all too often the patient will continue to be afflicted.

My approach to cystitis is to consider it in a far wider context. I try to find out why the patient has succumbed to the infection which has not apparently affected someone else. I look for the underlying cause or causes. I like my patients to know why their condition has developed, because an understanding helps the patients to help themselves.

Doctors far too frequently fail to explain things to their patients, and I suspect the reason is often that they don't know the explanation themselves and, of course, don't have the time. I don't just give a patient a pill and say 'Here! Take this. You should feel better in about a week or so.' Most of the patients I see have been through all that, and it either has not worked, or the treatment has given them side-effects.

To understand this book on cystitis, then, it will be helpful if the reader comes to understand my whole approach to medicine. My years as a medical student were spent at St. Bartholomew's Hospital in London. Most of what I was taught was based upon sound scientific knowledge and the experience of my forebears. Looking back on it today, I feel it left out areas of learning I would now consider of great value. Some of these are slowly entering the medical curricula of universities, but, because they have not been adequately explained from a scientific point of view, form only a minute part of a medical student's education.

After I qualified, I spent my first year at the Queen Elizabeth Hospital in Barbados, gaining at least five years' worth of experience in the one, doing things that few doctors of more than five years' experience are seldom allowed to do, let alone asked to do. Because there was no one else to do the work, I simply got on with it, and while my basic training had been comprehensive, it nowhere near covered what I had to do in Barbados. Often I simply had to improvise. It was this experience that made me start thinking of alternative ways of dealing with medical problems.

My next few years followed a more orthodox pattern, although a slightly unusual one for those days. I did some locums in general practice, worked in hospitals in anaesthetics, and obstetrics and gynaecology, gained postgraduate qualfications in both, and then joined Fisons, the pharmaceutical company. After doing some standard work required of a medical advisor, I helped start a department which experimented on humans, often on myself I might add, and I also took up a post as Honorary Clinical Assistant in the Department of Allergy at the Nottingham City Hospital.

One day, I came to treat a lady who felt that whenever she ate citrus fruits of any kind, even a small amount of lemon juice as seasoning, she would develop an urticarial rash (hives) 12 to 24 hours later. If she ate fish in any form, she would suffer terrible vomiting for the next 24 hours. She wanted to know if we could help her so that she would not need to avoid these foods. My work at that time at Fisons had involved investigating the action of a new drug called Intal®, which had been found to be capable of preventing asthmatic attacks when given by inhalation. In contrast to most of the drugs available at the time which simply treated the attack once the symptoms had started, Intal® was only useful if it was taken before an attack occurred. In other words it prevented the symptoms from developing. It occurred to me that if Intal® by inhalation could *prevent* an asthmatic attack, it might be possible also to prevent this lady's symptoms from occurring if she took some Intal® *by mouth* before eating the foods that made her ill. On a simple try-it-and-see basis, the idea worked. When put to the test properly in a special scientific way known as double-blind placebo-controlled, it also proved that Intal ® taken by mouth could block this woman's reactions.*

In the early 1970s hardly anyone knew anything about the way people reacted to certain items of their food, except for one man, Dr. Richard Mackarness. So I went down to the hospital in Basingstoke

**For full details of this report refer to the article 'Kingsley, P.J., Sodium Cromoglycate in Gastro-intestinal Allergy.' The Lancet*, 2: 1011, 1974.

where he had the first clinical ecology unit in Great Britain, and to my amazement, he opened my eyes to a way of treating patients that I had never seen before. (Clinical ecology is the study of Man's reaction to his environment, whether from what he eats, drinks, inhales or touches. It has been found that some people are made ill by a particular food, preservatives and additives, washing powders, lead in water pipes, even household pets.) It involved putting people onto strict diets, often a total fast for five days on bottled water only. This usually made them feel very well indeed and cleared their symptoms almost totally, suggesting that what they had previously been eating had been responsible for their ill health. He then fed them foods, one by one, that they had just avoided and found that some of these foods made them ill again, often the commonly eaten ones like milk, wheat, corn and sugar that no one had suspected. In this way he worked out a list of safe foods.

I visited Dr. Mackarness on a number of occasions and learned as much as I could from him before putting his ideas into practice in the Allergy Clinic at Nottingham City Hospital. In April 1977 I left Fisons after eight most interesting years and took over a rural general practice, where I treated as many patients as possible along the lines I had been learning.

A most important part of my training in clinical ecology was spent in Canada, where I lived for a short time with Dr. John McLennan near Toronto. To my mind he is the best and most practical teacher of clinical ecology I have had the pleasure to meet. He is still regularly teaching doctors in North America and is actively involved in the Society for Clinical Ecology, which has recently been renamed the American Academy of Environmental Medicine. Before the name change I was examined by Fellows of the Society and was made a Fellow in 1981.

In 1979, the British Clinical Ecology Group was formed under the guidance of Dr. George Hearn, Consultant Physician at the East Birmingham Hospital, and Dr. Ronald Finn, Consultant Physician at the Royal Liverpool Hospital. The original small group consisted of Drs. John Mansfield, Michael Radcliffe, Robin Husband, Richard Mackarness and myself. I was on the original committee and stayed on it when it was formally made into the British Society for Clinical Ecology in 1981. In December 1985, the name was changed to the British Society for Allergy and Environmental Medicine. Because of my commitment to clinical ecology, I not only lecture widely on this subject to professional and lay groups, but also run annual teaching weekends for medical practitioners.

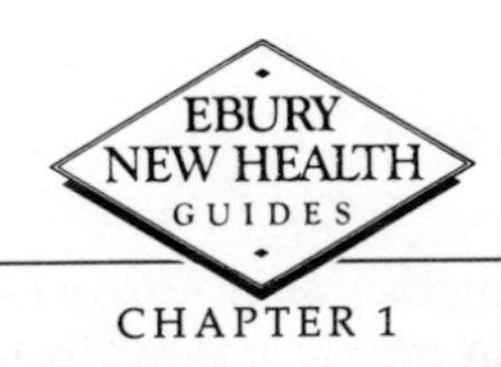

CHAPTER 1

THE AIMS OF THIS BOOK

RECURRENT or chronic cystitis, by their very names, suggest that attacks either don't go away properly, or seem to come back again too easily. This implies that either something is wrong with the treatment, or that a completely new approach is needed to prevent the next attack from developing. I hope to explain why the orthodox way of treating each attack with an antibiotic does not seem to work in the long run, and how changing your diet and certain other aspects of your life style will not only make you feel better but will cure your cystitis for good.

While a single attack of cystitis may well be caused by an infection, there has to be a reason why the problem comes back again. In some women there seem to be no obvious precipitating factors, while in other it seems to come on most commonly after sexual intercourse. A visit to the local doctor results in an antibiotic, which often provokes an attack of thrush, an irritant white curd-like vaginal dischange. This itself then needs appropriate treatment.

Why do some women get cystitis after intercourse and others do not, and why do some women develop thrush following the course of antibiotics and other do not? Even if they go through all the hospital tests, it is unusual for any explanation to be found. It is likely therefore that those who suffer have some predisposition towards cystitis, which, if found and removed, should stop the next attack from developing.

SEEKING THE UNDERLYING CAUSES

Cystitis is generally seen by doctors as a problem in the bladder, and its whole treatment concentrates on eliminating the symptoms from the bladder. This approach is a very narrow one. My explanation for recurrent cystitis is that something is 'irritating' the bladder, and that the *cause* has to be found and eliminated. By this means, the next attack will not occur. If sexual intercourse seems to precipitate an attack of cystitis, it suggests to me that there is some underlying mechanism being missed. The act of intercourse is surely the 'final straw'. I am more interested in what is making the camel's back weak in the first place. Commonly the load is either food allergies or candida albicans, the mould/yeast organism that is responsible for attacks of thrush. Whatever the cause, it must be traced and sorted out, so that intercourse can take place without cystitis being a frequent consequence.

I hope to be able to show people suffering from cystitis how to help themselves instead of relying on doctors, and how to be rid once and for all of those episodes of cystitis that sometimes occur out of the blue, only to settle and recur again for no apparent reason.

THE ORTHODOX APPROACH

Unfortunately, orthodox medicine sees cystitis as an entity on its own, and never really asks the question why it has happened. Medical education today is so confined to anatomy, physiology, pharmacology and the diagnosis of diseases and how they progress, that anything outside these concepts tends to be dismissed. What ordinary doctor would ever see a connection between a child kicking too much in the womb, a difficult two-week-late delivery, infantile colic, tonsillitis in infancy, the onset of heavy painful periods, pre-menstrual tension, an inability to tolerate the contraceptive pill, and cystitis? And yet there really is a link through them all, and indeed many other medical problems a patient may have suffered at some time in her life.

Despite an increasing number of women suffering form cystitis, the medical profession still blindly believes that treatment with drugs is the best and only form of management. The general attitude to patients is summed up by a story a medical colleague once told me. Many years ago he had worked with a general practitioner in Scotland, who said it was virtually pointless treating a patient when he or she first complained of something, unless, of course, it was one of those things that could not be ignored, like a heart attack, appendicitis, acute asthmatic attack, perforated eardrum etc. At the first presentation, he said, you should listen and be sympathetic but not too over-concerned, considering always whether this was just a ruse to visit the doctor about something far more personally important like a family row, which the patient could not bring him or herself to talk about once in the surgery.

When the patient came in again, after a suitable interval, this time complaining of something different, then it was likely there was a personal problem to sort out. If the patient complained of the same symptoms as when she first came in, the condition was likely to be genuine, said the old Scot. The third visit for the same complaint was to be taken seriously.

Because cystitis tends to be seen in simple terms (and possibly because a general practitioner's system of remuneration actually encourages him to give the patient as little time as he can get away with), each episode of cystitis is treated like the one before. Unless the doctor suffers from the same disease as the patient, he or she has little idea what the sufferer feels like. To many, many patients are attention-seekers and time-wasters, or sufferers from a psychosomatic disorder, which simply means their mind is causing, or possibly inventing, the physical symptoms. Unfortunately, most general practitioners, being male, have never suffered from cystitis and never will. They have no idea what cystitis feels like, no idea how much agony a woman can go through, especially as she *has* to pass water every so often. Cystitis tends to make you pass urine more often than normal, and the act of doing so can be agonizing.

From the descriptions some of my patients have given me of the pain of passing urine, the embarrassment of needing desperately to find a toilet, the worry passing blood can cause, and the havoc cystitis can cause with their marriage if sexual intercourse seems to be a major cause of the problem, there is little doubt in my mind how serious recurrent cystitis is.

For many patients the condition is intolerable, and can lead to thoughts of suicide. The regular pain it causes, the petrifying fear of the next attack, her inability to find anyone who can help, can all lead to severe depression. Imagine the guilt a man feels when he fears that every time he makes love to his wife she will soon be in agony again. How can any marriage survive that? Many do, but the rift between husband and wife gets ever greater.

Hope is raised for many patients by a referral to a specialist. Many visits, tests and examinations later, the patient is often no better. Indeed, some of the tests seem to bring the condition on. For many, antibiotics have the side-effects of a rash (the patient is then said to be allergic to that particular antibiotic), cause diarrhoea or indigestion, or may bring on a bout of thrush. The process a patient goes through under a specialist can be time consuming, often unpleasant, and in a very high percentage of cases, sadly ineffectual.

REFERRAL TO A PSYCHIATRIST

Cystitis is the bane of a urologist's life, just as irritable bowel syndrome is the gastroenterologist's. Many of his failures he refers to a psychiatrist which is, of course, appropriate only if the patient has become depressed.

Unfortunately, some psychiatrists have a field-day explaining how a woman who has symptoms of cystitis after sexual intercourse, is doing so deliberately as a ploy to stop her husband trying to make love to her, a typical Freudian theory, but one I totally reject. I firmly believe that most women who suffer from cystitis would dearly love to be free of their symptoms, free to live a normal life, and free to have normal sexual relations. By applying the methods outlined in this book, all of this is possible.

Recurrent cystitis is a condition causing distress to thousands of women every year, and clearly orthodox medicine is not being nearly helpful enough. Some women have periodic minor attacks of cystitis, some are frequently affected seriously. Some even have a constant feeling of pain or discomfort in the bladder area, with a degree of discomfort every time they pass urine.

While cystitis may be their main complaint, most of the women who have this awful condition will admit to other symptoms. It is far too easy to concentrate one's mind on the symptoms of cystitis, not realizing just how many other symptoms there may also be. In fact, pure chronic cystitis must be extremely rare. In general practice I certainly saw some women with their first attack of cystitis, who often said that they had had intercourse on a number of occasions over a special weekend, together with celebratory meals and more alcohol than usual. Others would appear to develop a single attack of cystitis without such a precipitating cause. A urine test and an appropriate antibiotic or other treatment would clear the symptoms well, and they would not be seen for the same condition again.

I once heard a helper from the Bristol Cancer Self-Help Group give a talk to the cancer self-help group that I am involved with locally. Her attitude was the same as mine. She described the time she was in hospital being investigated for cancer of her left breast, and found herself the subject of a particular teaching ward round. The specialist and all the doctors involved with him were only interested in her left breast; not the right, just the left one. They kept examining her left breast and talked about it all the time. With a degree of trepidation, she mentioned the headaches and nausea she regularly suffered, only to find them being dismissed as of no consequence at the time. The specialist said to her: 'We must deal with the cancer in your left breast first. Then, if necessary, we will think about the other problems.' He clearly didn't think that there could be any connection between them.

MY HOLISTIC APPROACH

My approach is different. For the first five minutes or so at an initial interview, I explain to the patient my attitude towards all ill health, describing the totally different concept I follow, and explaining how it differs from the orthodox view practiced by the vast majority of western doctors.

After discussing the main symptoms and talking all about them, I then ask for other problems, not just ones associated with cystitis. To start with, I let the patient slowly admit to a number of other unsatisfactory features, such as undue fatigue, periodic headaches, premenstrual irritation, episodes of weakness and hunger with cravings for sweets or chocolate, inability to cope and so on. Later, I ask specific questions, and it is amazing how many symptoms some people suffer from. They themselves are equally amazed that I should be interested in their whole body and not just their bladder. While cystitis is the main complaint, I am interested in the whole person.

I will explain why food allergies are likely to be the underlying cause of cystitis, and how they can be tracked down and treated. First, however, I will explain cystitis itself and the orthodox approach to it, and how the general practitioner and hospital specialist treat it. I will also describe some of the more specialized tests that look for an abnormality of structure and function.

THE AIMS OF THIS BOOK

The bulk of the book, however, will attempt to put across a completely different approach to trying to find the cause of the recurrent cystitis, concentrating on allergies to foods, indicating the importance of candida and thrush, and telling you how to unravel your own problems.

In each chapter I will explain how allergies develop, why the body fails to cope, and why cystitis may not be the only symptom affecting a person. In later chapters I go into considerable detail about how you can treat yourself, while Chapter Nine will basically be a summary of all the ideas put forward, with a thumbnail sketch of what to do.

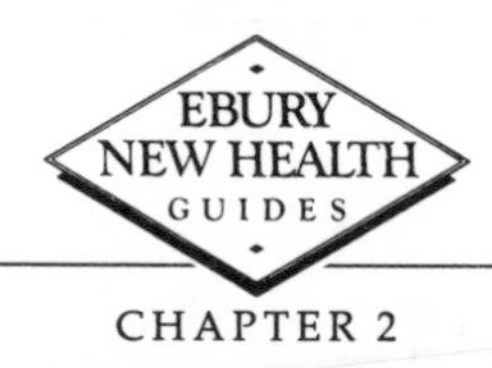

CHAPTER 2

CYSTITIS EXPLAINED

Cystitis means simply 'inflammation of the bladder'. Any word ending in 'itis' means inflammation, the first part of the word indicating the organ or area of the body that is inflamed, for example tonsill- itis, appendic- itis, arthr- itis. While a cyst is merely a sack, and can be used to indicate something quite harmless and small like a sebaceous cyst (a small fairly soft fluid-filled pebble-like structure under the skin or in the scalp), the 'cyst' in cystitis applies to the urinary bladder.

The Bladder and Urethra

Figure 1 shows the position of the bladder and urethra in a male, looking at him from the front, and figure 2 is that of the female. Figures 3 and 4 are male and female respectively, but a cross section viewed from the left side, in the middle of the body.

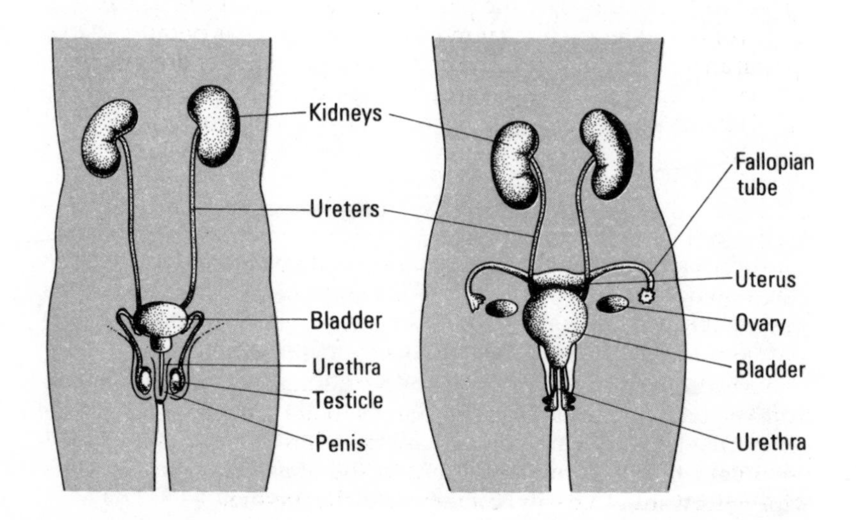

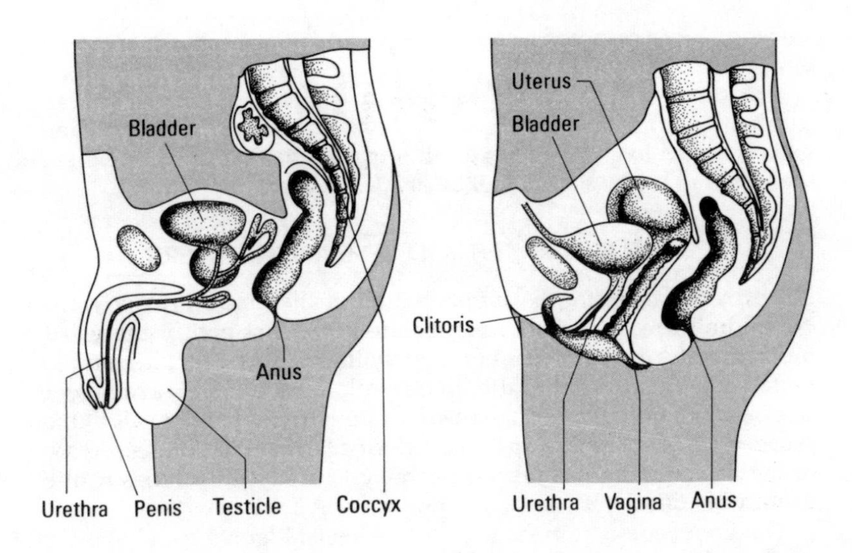

From these illustrations it is clear that the bladder (from which the word cystitis comes) is situated low in the abdomen, just above the pubis. This explains why the pain of cystitis is felt there. The reason why women suffer cystitis far more often than men is because of two special anatomical features. The first is the much shorter urethra in the female, making a much easier access for germs, if they are involved, to travel from the outside to enter the bladder. By looking at figure 3, what every woman probably knows yet may not have actually thought about, becomes obvious. That is, that she has three openings, the anus at the back, the vagina in the middle, and urethra at the front. In fact the vagina and urethra actually share a common opening of sorts, rather like two rivers entering the same bay before reaching the sea. The close proximity of the urethra to the vagina, and its near proximity to the anus, makes it distinctly possible for germs to pass from the vagina or anus to the urethra, and so lead to cystitis. Quite simply then, wiping the vagina or anus from the front backwards makes sense, rather than from the back forwards. Many infections in the urine are caused by a germ called Escherichia coli *(E. coli* for short), which is a regular inhabitant of the lower bowel and of the anus in particular. Thus wiping forward can easily 'contaminate' the urethra.

Candida is a common cause of cystitis and vaginal thrush (candida albicans is the mould/yeast organism that causes thrush), and is a common problem in women. Hence wiping the vagina forwards can 'contaminate' the urethra as well. Having said that, many women exercise good hygiene and still suffer from cystitis, and it is for these women that my approach will be of special value.

ANATOMY OF THE KIDNEYS AND URETERS

The ureters connect the bladder to the kidneys like two horns, although it is more correct to say that they connect the kidneys to the bladder, since urine flows from the kidneys to the bladder. The kidneys are situated at the back of the abdomen, and can be felt by an examining doctor's hands in the soft area between the bottom of the ribs at the back and the crest of the hip bone. A doctor can also sometimes feel the kidneys from in front. They are, however, buried inside the body by a number of other tissues and are not so easily felt.

The ureters pass from the kidneys to the bladder lying on the inner surface of the muscles at the back close to the spine, and when a stone gets stuck in a ureter it causes intense pain in the small of the back, in fact far worse than the pain of pyelitis. The pain of a stone starts off in spasms, but soon becomes continuous until the stone is passed.

SYMPTOMS OF CYSTITIS

Cystitis has a number of classic symptoms, some or all of which may be present.

Pain When Passing Urine

The most common symptom of cystitis is pain when passing urine. The degree of pain can vary enormously from a simple awareness that going to the toilet is accompanied by an altered sensation, through a feeling of burning or pain, to outright agony when urine flows through the channel leading from the bladder to the outside, the urethra. Various other phrases such as 'like passing hot coals' may be used by the patient to describe this pain, each one being descriptive and personal. The pain of cystitis should technically be confined to the bladder itself, and will therefore be in the lower part of the abdomen above the pubic bone (see figure 1). In fact, a diagnosis of cystitis is most commonly made when there is some degree of pain on passing urine, which should therefore more strictly be called urethritis. Pain on passing urine is the symptom most commonly complained of when the patient is said to have cystitis, and if the patient tells her G.P. she has cystitis, he or she will most likely assume her main or only symptom is pain on passing water.

If directly questioned, the patient may say she has pain in her lower abdomen on passing water, or may describe it as 'a bearing down sensation', but the urethritis is the main symptom.

Volume of Urine

Because the bladder is irritated, the muscles in its wall tend to contract so that the bladder does not seem to be capable of holding as much urine as normal. This results in the patient passing urine more often than normal, but in smaller amounts. The sensation of 'wanting to go' is governed by stretch receptors in the wall of the bladder, so that as soon as the bladder wall is stretched by urine filling it, a sense of desire to go to the toilet results. Even when the bladder wall is in spasm because of the irritation, the same seems to apply. However, the bladder is seldom emptied as much in cystitis as it is in health, and, even though the patient finishes urinating, she often feels that she is not quite empty but cannot seem to squeeze out any more. It is the inflammation in the bladder wall that produces this sensation.

Sometimes, although it is not obvious when, the bladder stays the normal size, and can fill up with the usual amount of urine. This is less common, but means the patient is not passing urine quite so often as other sufferers from cystitis. In these cases, the residual urine (i.e. the amount still left when finished urinating) may be that much more. If it is infected, this makes it all the more likely that infection will creep up towards the kidneys.

Passing Blood

When it first occurs, the passing of blood in the urine can be most alarming, and at times a lot of blood can be passed. There is no known reason why some people bleed when others don't, but I have found it interesting that a high percentage of cystitis bleeders (if you will pardon the expression!) also feel they bruise more easily than seems reasonable. I believe this may well be a deficiency of vitamin K, although Prothombin Time Tests (the normal test of blood clotting that is used as a screening test for any bleeding tendency) are always normal when I have had them done. The reason for the Vitamin K deficiency may well be the presence of candida and other yeast/moulds in the intestine, a subject which will be covered more fully in Chapter Six.

Some patients bleed so much they actually start to feel faint, although some faint just at the sight of blood. However, the pain of cystitis is enough to cause faintness. Occasionally, the blood loss can be sufficient actually to cause anaemia, which in any case tends to be a problem in women because of their monthly blood loss through their periods. It is my observation that patients who bleed with cystitis tend to have heavier and more painful periods, which again tends to be more common when candida is present. What I find so fascinating is how all these observations tie up, and can often be explained. When cystitis is treated by the methods to be outlined in this book, many patients find their periods also improve, as well as their premenstrual tension. Almost always, other symptoms disappear as well.

Raised Temperature

When the bladder and urethra only are inflamed, it is unusual to have a raised temperature. If a fever does occur it almost always means that the urine has become infected by a virus or germ, but it does not necessarily mean that antibiotics are appropriate, since they are of no value against viruses. Indeed in many attacks of cystitis, an infection is undoubtedly involved though it is not neccessarily the cause, and yet there is no fever. If fever does occur, it is usually a sign that the infection has spread outside the bladder and urethra towards the kidneys.

Spread into the Kidneys

Doctors talk mainly of cystitis and occasionally of urethritis, but they never talk of ureteritis (inflammation of the ureters down which urine flows from the kidneys to the bladder). This is strange because when the infection in the urine pooled in the bladder spreads towards the kidneys, it is the collecting area that becomes involved, which is called pyelitis. If it goes into the kidneys it is known as pyelo-nephritis, whilst chronic inflammation of the kidneys is simply called nephritis. As the glomeruli of the kidney (where urine is first made by filtration from the blood) may be inflamed, the term glomerulo-nephritis is available to doctors, but a diagnosis can really only be made by looking at a sample (biopsy) of the kidney under a microscope.

Although pyelitis and nephritis are not really within the scope of this book, anyone who has these problems could do themselves a power of good by following some of the ideas presented here, for it is important to realize that chronic infections in the bladder can lead to chronic infections in the kidneys. Strangely enough, however, most cases of chronic nephritis do not start with obvious cystitis. Many doctors therefore feel that women should have a regular urine check since they feel that chronic nephritis develops as a result of unrecognized silent urine infections. I find that an implausible theory, but cannot prove they are wrong. I feel it is merely another symptom of something wrong somewhere with the body.

PAIN OF PYELITIS

Apart from the fever already mentioned, there is pain in the loin area of the back when cystitis has spread to become pyelitis. The pain can, in fact, be very bad indeed, and what with the pain in the lower abdomen from the cystitis and the burning of passing urine, the patient can be in a very bad way. Although the theme of this book is the management of cystitis without drugs, I would never doubt the wisdom of using antibiotics and pain killers once pyelitis has developed.

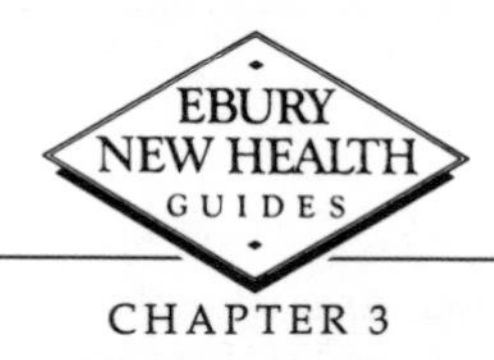

CHAPTER 3

THE ORTHODOX APPROACH

Because doctors don't believe in food and chemical allergies, it never occurs to them that they could cause a patient's cystitis. To be fair, I suppose it has never occurred to most doctors that cystitis could be caused by an allergy – they were never taught such an idea in their medical training, they never hear it suggested at postgraduate lectures, and they have not read about the idea in their educational and promotional literature. No pharmaceutical company is going to encourage such a prospect, since looking for a food cause will not encourage a doctor to prescribe the company's drugs.

Most doctors assume that cystitis is caused by an infection in the urine. The only reason a doctor sometimes has the patient's urine specimen examined by the local laboratory is to check that a bacterium (germ) is responsible rather than a virus, as antibiotics are of no value in viral infections, and to find out which antibiotic to give. A recent paper published in October 1985 in the *British Medical Journal* is entitled 'Staphylococcus Saprophyticus as a Urinary Pathogen; A Six Year Prospective Study.' Quite clearly, doctors are still looking for specific infections as a cause of cystitis.

As doctors are aware of 'honeymoon cystitis', they know that a woman's current trouble could be intercourse, possibly too frequent or too active intercourse. Once the urethra has become inflamed, a germ may invade the damaged tissue and set up an infection, so the patient will most likely be given an antibiotic. It is assumed that, if an antibiotic happens not to be needed it won't do any harm.

With the occasional episode of cystitis, most doctors will prescribe an appropriate antibiotic, with or without a urine test first. It is a general practitioner's experience that women tend to suffer from cystitis anyway, so it is a major part of his or her practice to see women with this condition. When the condition occurs more often than he thinks is reasonable (a very arbitrary situation), or if the symptoms are very severe or the condition involves the kidneys, he will refer the patient to the local specialist for advice.

Because the cystitis has now become a bit of a problem to the patient, and because he may be unhappy at prescribing too many antibiotics too frequently the G.P. wonders if there may be a cause which requires further investigation. By now he has presumably done a urine test and examined the patient, and not been able to explain to himself why the condition keeps coming back. He therefore suspects there might be 'something wrong' with the bladder, such as a congenital malformation or a sinus.

CONGENITAL MALFORMATION

Some people are born with an extra finger, a hare lip, short arms (as caused by thalidomide) or something of that sort which may or may not cause trouble in life. Occasionally an investigating specialist will find that the patient has an extra ureter on one side, or on both sides, i.e. has three or four ureters instead of the normal two. Most of the time these cause no trouble whatsoever, but on occasions one of them may not connect properly with the bladder, there may be a constriction or a blind tube.

When a blind tube is found, it is assumed that urine stagnates there and becomes infected. On its own the urine in it should remain sterile even if it is stagnant, but, once the urine in the bladder has become infected, some of the infected urine may remain in the blind tube. When antibiotics pass down the ureters from the kidney to the bladder, they may not mix properly with the stagnant urine, and so a continuous source of infection is set up. This may be partially cleared up by the antibiotics, but, as the germs there are not properly and completely killed, a form resistant to that antibiotic may well develop. It will require another urine test to find out which antibiotic is now needed.

If the urine in the stagnant pool does not initially become infected, crystals may form and enlarge into 'stones'. These may irritate the lining of the tube and lead to simple inflammation. The wall at the end of the tube may therefore swell so that the opening into the bladder becomes blocked. The wall of the bladder near the extra tube opening will also become inflamed, but may never become infected. It is possible therefore that constant bladder inflammation may result, which will lead to persistent low abdominal pain or discomfort, defying all explanation until the surgeon has a look inside or does some other tests.

If an infection does occur in conjunction with such a congenital malformation it is easy to see how the infection can be perpetuated, how it may be difficult to eradicate, why a resistant form of germ may subsequently be found, and why recurrent cystitis will develop. It must be appreciated, however, that a malformation is not a common cause of chronic cystitis.

SINUS

A sinus is a tube that leads from one organ to another, that should not be there, but which has developed as a result of some other condition. It most commonly arises in Crohn's Disease and in inflammation of the bowel. As certain parts of the bowel lie close to or on the bladder, inflammation of one of those parts of the bowel may involve the bladder as well. They therefore become stuck to each other. If too large an area of both bladder and bowel become inflamed together, the blood supply to the central part is cut off and becomes necrotic (dies). Eventually the dead cells break away and a communication develops between the bladder and bowel interiors. More commonly, however, the bowel inflammation merely causes inflammation of the bladder wall itself, with all the problems already described.

Whichever happens, germs from the bowel find their way more easily into the bladder and set up cystitis. The common germ is *E. coli*. Despite eradication with a course of antibiotics, it is all too easy to see how recurrent infections of the bladder occur.

VISITING THE SPECIALIST AND HAVING TESTS

When the specialist sees the patient for the first time, he is likely to start from scratch. He will ask as many questions as reasonable to throw light upon the possible causes, such as 'Does your cystitis occur after intercourse?' 'Do you pass blood in your urine?' He will also ask a number of other questions that seem relevant to him.

He will then examine you all over, concentrating not just on your bladder area. He will take your blood pressure, more of a sensible routine than expecting a raised blood pressure to have anything to do with a current problem of cystitis. He will arrange for another urine test, and will expect the outpatient sister or nurse to explain to the patient how to take it properly. Occasionally a sterile catheter will be inserted through the urethra into the bladder if the opening of the urethra looks contaminated already.

CYSTOSCOPY

If the severity of the patient's condition justifies it, and if in his opinion the condition appears to be confined to the bladder, he will arrange for the patient to have a cystoscopy. This is a simple procedure (to the surgeon), in which he inserts an instrument called a cystoscope (a scope to use on the bladder – the *cyst*) through the urethra into the bladder. The patient will be under a light general anaesthetic, as it can be rather uncomfortable, but will probably be allowed home later that day.

Under the anaesthetic the surgeon will have a good look round inside the bladder. The cystoscope has a light on the end of it and tubes which allow water to be passed into the bladder to wash it out. Usually another urine sample is taken first as the procedure for inserting the cystoscope is completely sterile. Therefore any infection in the sample should have come from the urine inside the bladder rather than be a contamination of the sample during the taking of it. Flushing the bladder out with sterile water gives the surgeon a good view of the wall, and he can look all round to see if there are any growths, protrusions, indentations, areas of inflammation, or anything that appears to be unusual to his experienced eye. He will also examine the entrance into the bladder from the ureters to check that they are not only normal-looking, but also that there are only two of them!

I.V.P.

If the surgeon feels it is called for, he will arrange for an I.V.P. (an intravenous pyelogram) to be carried out by a colleague in the radiology department. This is unlikely to be arranged for the same day, unless the patient has been admitted for extensive investigations. It is more likely to be organized on an outpatient basis and done on another day.

A dye will be injected into a vein in the arm and a plain X-ray will be taken of the abdominal area. After a suitable time to allow the dye to circulate in the blood and be excreted in the kidneys, other X-rays will be taken which will outline the kidneys and show clearly the structure of the tubes that collect the urine coming out of the body of the kidney.

Later X-rays will show the structure of the ureters, how many there are, and whether there is any abnormality. Their position on entering the bladder will be checked and, when the bladder is full of the contrast medium (the dye), pressure will be applied to the lower abdomen to look for any reflux back up the ureters from the bladder. The anatomical arrangement at the junction of ureters and bladder should prevent any urine passing back up the ureters, but, when it does occur, it is considered a possible malfunctioning cause of cystitis. The dye shows the smoothness or otherwise of the wall of the bladder and whether there are any obstructions, pockets or pouches.

Depending upon the results of all these tests, the specialist will decide what to do. Despite the fact that the vast majority of these special X-ray tests and operations will be normal, it is important that they be done once to make sure there is not an underlying problem that can explain it all. If there is a congenital malformation of the ureters, or a wart or other growth on the bladder wall, they should be dealt with in the appropriate way. Warty growths and congenital malformations need a surgeon's skill.

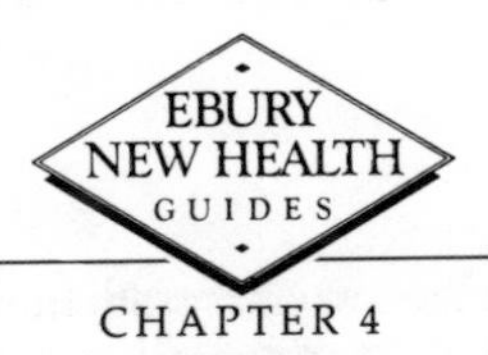

CHAPTER 4

MY ALTERNATIVE APPROACH

THE orthodox approach to all disease, including problems with the bladder, is that the organ that is showing symptoms is what is at fault. In the case of cystitis, the bladder or urethra are at fault and the problem is assumed to be the bladder or its wall or contents. Orthodox doctors concentrate on the bladder and its surroundings, all the time looking for something there to explain the symptoms. Keep looking and eventually, they think, they will find the cause in the bladder. When they do they can either operate on it or give the patient a drug to treat the bladder.

I have deliberately repeated the word 'bladder' in the last paragraph in order to explain the blinkered approach to cystitis of the majority of doctors. This is what they believe, what they teach and what they practice, despite the fact that this approach seldom does the patient much good. Admittedly, the occasional attack of cystitis may appear to respond to a course of antibiotics, but often it will go away anyway even if it is not treated. The time it takes to go away often corresponds to the time it would have taken for the antibiotic to kill an infection, if it had been the cause.

Because this approach all too often meets with failure, it amazes me that doctors stick to it. Why don't they look for other ways of explaining it, and thereby help their poor suffering patients? Could it be that they don't need to get their patients better because their reputation does not depend upon success? That may be rather a cynical question and I hope it is wrong. Nevertheless, there must be some reason for this narrow approach that fails so often. After all, doctors are intelligent people. The exams they have to pass prove that. Could it be that since they have to read so much written by their forebears and teachers that they have little time for real thinking of their own? They have to follow the established way or they won't pass their exams and progress up the medical ladder. Perhaps the system indoctrinates them.

Let us now step back and view the body as a whole, and make an assumption that the body has a natural inbuilt ability to be normal, and a natural desire to become normal again if it has temporarily become abnormal. If you were born with a structural deformity, I don't know of any way we can yet do anything about it. If you were born without an arm, medicine knows of no way to make that arm grow to become a normal arm with a hand and fingers that work properly. We can try to fashion an artificial limb, but it will never be a real one.

When the majority of patients present to their doctor or the hospital specialist, nothing is found to be wrong with them – structurally or functionally, that is. But there must be something wrong or else the patient wouldn't be complaining. Yet the doctor cannot find what it is. All too often he gives up and puts it down to 'nerves', or says it is 'all in the mind'.

Because the body will function normally in ideal circumstances, if it is starting to go wrong the circumstances for normal operating must somehow have become abnormal. The environment in which the body is trying to work correctly has somehow become 'poisoned' or is not quite right. The environment of the body is the air breathed in, the food eaten, the water drunk, the surroundings the body comes into contact with, the stresses of everyday life that become too much for it to cope with, the pollution imposed by petrol and diesel fumes, the chemicals in our food and homes. It is these we must look to to find the reasons why our bodies are going wrong. *It is the environmental causes that the sufferer from chronic cystitis must investigate to help herself.*

Let us take two examples to illustrate this further. You set out in your car one cold morning, pulling out the choke as you start it. Inadvertently you leave the choke out all the way to town, the car starts to play up on you, you think there is something wrong with the engine, and you blame the garage for not having serviced it properly. Then you realize you have left the choke out. You push it in and gradually the engine returns to normal. There was nothing wrong with the engine. It was the environment for normal functioning that was incorrect.

As another example, imagine being exposed to C.S. anti-riot gas which is designed to incapacitate people. Mucus is produced in response to the gas and the eyes not only sting and smart, they also run so that you cannot see what you are doing. Your nose pours and it is also uncomfortable. In your lungs the gas causes irritation so that you start to cough violently and produce a lot of phlegm. Your skin smarts. It is not surprising that C.S. gas is efficient at controlling crowds for nearly everyone who is exposed to it is affected. It is a toxic substance to all humans, so it is not really an allergic substance, as an allergy is something specific to you, and does not necessarily affect anyone else.

The symptoms in your eyes, nose, lungs and skin are caused by the poisoned environment. They cannot function properly because the environment has been made abnormal. When the gas clears in the wind and fresh air returns, the symptoms begin to settle and, within a reasonable length of time, you return to normal.

No one blames your eyes, nose, lungs and skin, saying they are responsible for the symptoms. No one does fancy tests to see what is wrong with them, to try to find out why they are behaving so badly. No one passes a tube into your lungs to find what is wrong with them to see why they are producing so much mucus. No one takes a sample of your skin to see why it is smarting. The explanation is all too obvious. It is the irritant effect of the C.S. gas.

What I am trying to do is make a point. Symptoms are produced not because the organ is at fault, but because something in it's environment has made it react. In the case of cystitis, it is true that an infection can be involved or is occasionally the cause, but in so many people it just does not explain why they are ill and why their cystitis keeps coming back.

It is important that a person suffering from chronic or recurrent cystitis has a number of tests done, but when they have failed to explain the cause a search in a far wider context should be made. The doctor should consider whether food or chemical allergies are at fault, and either investigate the possibility himself or ask a colleague to do it who is interested and experienced in these techniques.

Everyone knows their stomach and intestines can be upset by eating the wrong food. Surely, therefore, it is perfectly reasonable to suggest that cystitis may be caused by something put into the bladder, in the urine. In fact cystitis can result from something being carried in the blood stream ending in the wall of the bladder and setting up a reaction.

THE TARGET ORGAN

What is not clear is why a particular part of the body becomes the target of an allergy. Why don't all organs react? Do we have weak spots in our system? Are we born with some congenital tendency that makes our liver, our skin, our brain, or our bladder, for example, react adversely when other organs of the body don't? It would be nice to know the answer to this question, but quite frankly it doesn't really matter. What is important is to find out *what* is causing the problem and deal with it in the appropriate way.

Certainly, the sooner the cause is found and dealt with the easier it is. If the condition has been going on for 30 to 40 years, you cannot expect it to go away overnight. Once the cause has been tracked down the body has a lot of hard work to do to return to normal functioning. In those 30 to 40 years, a lot of changes will have taken place, all of which have to be corrected in their turn.

Imagine a builder being asked to renovate a historic building that has been left empty for 30 to 40 years. Damp, corrosion, mould, the lot have eaten into the fabric of the house. The pipes are all rusty and will have to be replaced. The roof will need to be re-done, plaster replaced, new wallpaper and paint applied. Plants growing wildly on the outside will have to be removed and the brickwork will have to be repaired, replaced or re-pointed. The garden will need a lot of work. I am sure you see the analogy with the human body.

For this reason, children tend to be very easy to treat. Their response to treatment is usually simple, rapid and highly rewarding. Fortunately, cystitis is seldom suffered by children. On the other hand, cystitis in an adult is often the accumulation of a number of problems that have been inadequately dealt with over the years. Occasionally a person starts to suffer from cystitis, having until recently been in good health. All too often, however, there has been something wrong on and off for some time, and now cystitis is the main problem troubling the patient. At times it is one of a number of concurrent complaints.

While it may be difficult or impossible to explain why a particular part of the body such as the skin, lungs or joints are now the target organ for the ill health, it is quite possible there may be acceptable reasons why the bladder is so frequently affected. It is basically the same reason why the intestines so frequently play up. It is often what goes into them that is important.

As I firmly believe that what people eat can affect their health and produce symptoms, what goes into the intestines is of vital importance. Not surprisingly, foods and drinks can affect the intestines themselves, the upper part of the bowel being mainly affected by what is put into it. The lower part, the colon in particular, is affected by what is left after the process of digestion and absorption. While eating foods a person is allergic to may cause symptoms, leaving out others can also do harm. It is well recognized that if the bowel does not have enough fibre to stimulate it, constipation will result. Without vitamins and minerals in the diet, nutritional deficiencies will occur.

The corollary with the bladder should be obvious. Urine is considered to be waste from the body, but in fact it is the body's most efficient method of getting rid of what it does not want. There are many breakdown products of metabolism, but if they were taken back into the body, the system would re-use what it wanted at the time and excrete the rest. Urine certainly contains substances the body does not want to retain, substances the body wants to get rid of. It may also contain substances that the greater part of the body can tolerate, only to find that the bladder itself cannot tolerate them. Hence cystitis develops.

When a person starts developing diabetes, sugar accumulates in the body, and to a certain extent the body can tolerate a degree of excess. The kidneys have a threshold, however, and when it is exceeded sugar is spilled over into the urine. Because sugar is hypertonic (i.e. is basically thicker than the serum of the blood) more water has to be excreted to dissolve the sugar and keep the urine thin and flowing. Nevertheless, the urine of a diabetic tastes sweet, hence the name diabetes mellitus (from the Latin word *mel* meaning honey).

As every doctor knows, one of the first signs of diabetes is passing excessive amounts of urine (to dissolve the sugar). Because he knows this connection between frequent micturition (passing water very often) and diabetes, he does not examine the bladder. He merely confirms that sugar is being passed into the urine. He then gives dietary advice to reduce the amount of sugar taken in the diet, and suggests injections of insulin if they are called for. When the treatment begins to work, the urinary problems start to settle.

With diabetes in mind, you can see the reasoning behind my 'alternative' approach to cystitis. As with diabetes, the symptoms of cystitis are caused by something wrong some way off from the bladder itself. When the causes are found and dealt with, the presenting symptoms disappear. There are so many examples of this that it makes me despair when doctors say this approach is all nonsense, simply because it is not what they were taught. The results speak for themselves. It is almost impossible to turn on the television or radio without some condition being discussed along these lines. The sadness is that the people qualified to manage the treatment of these poor patients don't seem to know about it!

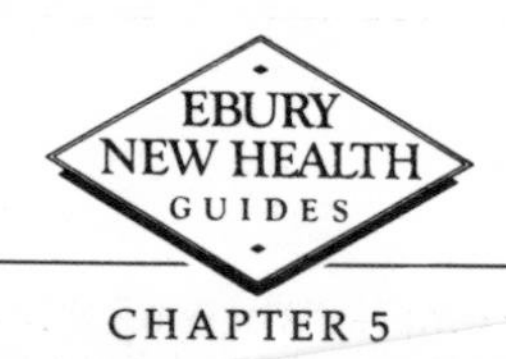

CHAPTER 5

UNDERSTANDING ALLERGIES AND ADDICTIONS

I LIKE my patients to understand why their bodies have started complaining. Whenever possible I try to take time to give a full explanation of all my observations, but, within the time constraints of an hour's consultation, it is invariably incomplete. This chapter will put the whole process into perspective, and if each patient reading it will consider what is being said in relation to herself, I am sure the picture will become clear. In parts she will probably say 'That's me to a tee!'. In other areas, she will not find the idea so appropriate. Remember, everyone is an individual, we are all different and we will react differently, even if there is a common theme.

It is my belief that food or chemical allergies are the cause of recurrent cystitis in many women. It is my hope that by reading this book and putting certain of the advice into practice, each sufferer will be able not only to track down the cause, but also eliminate it, and thereby not suffer from cystitis.

The word 'allergy' means different things to different people, but when it was originally invented by von Pirquet in 1906, he simply meant 'a state of reactivity', or quite simply 'a reaction'. In the early part of this century the science of medicine was far less precise than it is today, and the mechanism by which an allergy caused symptoms was not known.

ALLERGISTS AND IMMUNOLOGISTS

Immunologists, however, have adopted the word allergy to mean something special. Various chemical and biological pathways involving immunoglobulins, T-helper cells, T-suppressor cells, B-cells and leukotrienes, etc., have all been identified, and the mechanisms of allergic reactions established. Thus, to the medical scientist, the word 'allergy' should be confined to a reaction in which a specific immunological pathway has been established, or can be demonstrated in a particular patient.

Frequently, a patient complains of something and is investigated by an allergist or immunologist, only to find that the tests do not prove that the patient is allergic. He or she may have suspected that egg was the cause of their symptoms, and wanted confirmation by an appropriate specialist. With any luck, the tests confirm the patient's suspicions and an appropriate diet is recommended. Often they do not. This leaves the patient in a quandary, especially if he is sure in his own mind that eggs are responsible.

Strictly speaking, the immunologist is probably right, but only in a pedantic, narrow way. By saying the patient is 'not allergic' to eggs, he is merely indicating that if a reaction is being caused by eggs, it is not an allergy in the sense that he understands it because it does not follow the established immunological pathways. The orthodox doctor is inclined to believe the patient to be wrong in his observations, it never occurring to him that the patient may be right and that he, the doctor, is the one who is wrong.

Many reactions to foods are indeed an allergic response but the majority of reactions do not follow the established immunological line. Some other mechanism, as yet to be established, is involved. Kinin-inflammatory mechanisms are one alternative, and terms such as hypersensitivity or idiosyncrasy may be used.

To the orthodox immunologist an allergic reaction means that the body's defence mechanisms (immune system) are over-responding to a particular challenge by an allergen (a substance that provokes an allergic reaction).

When the body is first exposed to a potential allergen, it produces antibodies against it, but for reasons that are not understood, it produces too many on subsequent exposure. As a result, symptoms develop. Treatment is either aimed at dampening down the over-production of antibodies or stopping them resulting in symptoms.

Avoidance of the allergen is also advantageous but can be extremely difficult to achieve. Helmets with filtered air have been devised for use in the hay fever season, but most people feel too self-conscious and therefore won't leave home in one. They are therefore likely to accept having to be exposed to grass pollen in summer.

To most doctors an allergy, then, is not only something highly specific and has a demonstrable pathway, but is specific to that person. The press and general public have adopted the word allergy to mean any reaction whatever the cause. Emotive terms such as 'allergic to the twentieth century' and ' the total allergy syndrome' have been banner headlines in some newspapers.

In practical terms an allergy, however it is defined, is an individual's reaction to something. It is the individual's personal response, and the fact that he or she responds to it and others do not is something to do with his or her make-up and present state of health.

By and large allergic reactions are considered to be limited to certain symptoms. Hay fever is an established allergic disease which causes symptoms of a runny nose with sneezing, eyes that are itchy, sore and runny, and sometimes asthma. An allergy to house dust, animal dander, flowers, etc., can produce the same symptoms all the year round. Allergic skin reactions are eczema (dry, itchy, weeping skin) and urticaria (in which lumps or rashes of various sizes develop). Swellings of the mouth, lips, tongue, breathing tubes, etc., are acknowledged allergic reactions to fish and eggs. Diarrhoea and vomiting may be the result of an allergic reaction to shell fish in a susceptible person.

Outside these reactions, it is seldom considered that an allergy could be involved. If the doctor were to examine his patients closely, he would also find other symptoms being complained of, but which tend to be ignored. The hay fever sufferer often complains of loss of ability to concentrate, temporarily reduced memory and depression, even if he is not on anti-histamines which can cause drowsiness as well. The patient who has diarrhoea and vomiting from eating shell fish often complains of terrible aching in his joints. An asthmatic may develop a headache or indigestion.

HOW ALLERGIES DEVELOP

Basic to an understanding of the whole concept of allergies is a knowledge of how they develop, how the symptoms may become masked, and how addictions develop. It is therefore worthwhile briefly describing the original work done by Hans Selye, Professor of Experimental Medicine and Surgery at the University of Montreal.*

In 1936 Selye published a short account of experimental work in animals, in which he stressed them in various ways, for example, with heat, cold and toxic substances, and watched the effect. In 1946 he added allergens to his list of stressor factors. He found that all living organisms responded in the same three-stage way. Stage one was alarm, like surgical shock: stage two was recovery, going into a phase

* *Selye, H. 'The General Adaption Syndrome and the Diseases of Adaptation.' American Journal of Allergy, 17, 1946.*

of resistance or adaptation after a few days if the stressing agent was continually applied; and stage three (much later), a phase of exhaustion, from which they did not survive because of pituitary and adrenal exhaustion. While Selye placed relatively greater emphasis on the general features of adaptation, it was Professor Adolph of New York who reported in 1956 similar responses, but had found that individual animals showed marked differences in their response to the same stressor, and that the effect of that stressor could be different under different conditions. He was thus proposing in animals what we know to be true in man – each person is an individual.

In stage one, a single application of a stressor (something which is capable of doing any sort of harm to the body) produces recognizable symptoms, from which recovery should be complete. If that stressor is applied at wide intervals, it will always cause the same symptoms unless the amount of stress is considerably increased, in which case additional symptoms may occur.

If the stressor is applied again just as recovery has been achieved, and then repeated at regular short-spaced intervals, it will induce an adaptive response which may actually give a feeling of well being, instead of producing unpleasant symptoms; the alarm reaction described by Hans Selye. By developing 'pleasant' instead of unpleasant symptoms, the person has entered a new phase of reactivity – stage two.

In stage two, the person tends to feel well all the time, although the occasional dip in health can occur for no obvious reason. The sense of well-being is maintained by the stressor being constantly applied, like a food to which they have become allergic being eaten regularly. Theoretically this good feeling in stage two could go on forever, because the human organism (human being) is a very adaptable creature. Most people would agree that humans thrive on interest, which is a comfortable stimulus. When that interest is overdone it becomes a stress. Even then, a human can take a reasonable amount of stress for quite a long time – but not forever without paying a price.

In stage two, a dip in the sense of well being can be caused by temporarily stopping eating a food to which the person's body has become tolerant without realizing it. As soon as he starts eating that food again he get back to where he was before. Actually, the dip may be only a recognition of the difference between being 'too well' and getting somewhere near the normal line. Because a pendulum has a habit of swinging beyond the mid line, the patient may actually not feel at all well. To someone else this may be only a minor degree of feeling not so well, but to him the contrast is so great he feels worse than he really ought.

If the person in stage two were to be questioned deeply and compared with so-called normal people, things would be found to be not so perfect. He may well be just a bit agitated, plan to do things that are impractical and which are never completed even if they are started. At first sight such people seem outgoing, devil-may-care, the main attraction of the evening. When you get to know them they are a bit headstrong, arrogant, bossy and not too reliable. All too easily they become has-beens. There are two main reasons why the organism may start failing to adapt, i.e. change from stage two to stage three. The first is that the stressor may be a very strong one, or there may be more than one. The second reason is that an additional stressor may be applied in the form of a bereavement, an operation or an accident, etc. In nearly all cases this causes the person to change his or her dietary habits, usually for the worse at a time when nutritional excellence is vital. Nutritional deficiencies will therefore occur and not give the body's homoeostatic mechanisms a chance to recover.

Stress in any form produces a considerably increased requirement for many vitamins and minerals, notably zinc, vitamin C and the B vitamins. If their intake has been inadequate or only just adequate before the extra stress factor, the chances are that they will not only be insufficient to cover the stress, but their intake will actually go down at the time of the stressful event. That additional stress is therefore bound to have a disastrous effect. When taking a history, it is amazing how often symptoms seem to the patient to have started a short time after a particular event, nearly always a stressful one. In some it can be what are considered normal life events, such as childbirth or moving house.

Whatever the reason for the person's adaptive mechanisms starting to fail, stage three is the beginning of the downhill trek, when symptoms become a nuisance again, and when they tend to be more persistent. While specific symptoms such as arthritis, migraine and colitis may start troubling patients, to begin with there may be more minor symptoms such as unreasonable fatigue, inability to lose weight, inability to sleep, depression, odd headaches and agitation.

Sudden episodes of really not feeling at all well, dizziness, light-headedness, sweating and a sense of hunger may well develop, especially when the person is hungry or shortly before meals. They notice they can make themselves better by having a bar of chocolate, a cup of sweet tea or coffee, or just something to eat (usually a carbohydrate food). This is hypoglycaemia, and will be discussed in

Chapter Six, but it is also a clear sign the adaptive mechanisms are failing and that the body can no longer handle the large amounts of carbohydrate consumed throughout that person's life.

It can be seen then that any substance, be it a food, drink, chemical, drug, etc., can induce different symptoms according to which stage the patient is in. In stage one, symptoms only occur when the patient is exposed to that substance. If the symptoms are clearly related in time by the patient, that substance tends to be avoided. Such obvious reactions are a rash from eating strawberries in summer or too much chocolate at Easter, diarrhoea and vomiting after eating shell fish, or a migraine caused by cheese, chocolate or red wine.

Unfortunately, however, most patients fail to recognize what is causing the symptoms. It simply does not occur to them. In addition, the onset of symptoms may be some hours after eating food, therefore making it difficult to blame that food. Sadly the fact that foods could be causing the patient's symptoms is unknown to their doctor.

In fact, the first evidence of a stage one reaction may be in infancy, when the child has colic, eczema or unreasonable upper respiratory problems, whether being breast or bottle fed. On occasions a mother may recognize that her baby becomes hyperactive or peaceful in the womb according to what she herself eats. Far too often these first stage one signs are ignored. When the child is weaned symptoms may appear to settle, largely because the offending food is now taken in smaller amounts as other foods are introduced into the child's diet.

In stage two, there may be no easily recognized symptoms, although if the substance is temporarily stopped, there may be a sudden loss of energy and even a mildly depressed phase. As soon as the substance is taken in again, so long as the gap is not too great, say three days, the patient will get right back to where he was. Thus the allergy is being masked. Constant exposure to the allergenic food is masking the fact that the patient *needs* it regularly. So long as he continues to eat it, as he most likely will, he could remain comfortably in stage two for the rest of his life, unless something happens to make him enter stage three.

In stage three, he unconsciously realizes that he needs more of a particular substance to maintain his previous state of well-being. As the body's adaptive mechanisms begin to fail, the 'pick-me-up' effect of an exposure to that substance does not last so long, nor is it as effective as it used to be. To maintain the 'good' feeling the patient needs a bigger dose more often. He is becoming un-masked and is on the addictive merry-go-round.

Once stage three is properly established, the patient is unwell much of the time. Symptoms certainly occur on avoidance, and become more severe on avoidance as stage three progresses. Clearly the pattern of addiction has now been established, but it is amazing how the food and cigarette addict doesn't compare himself to the alcohol or hard drug addict. Despite recognizing that he now 'needs' his sugar, coffee or cigarettes, his symptoms on withdrawal are so bad that he cannot imagine life without them. He does not realize they are killing him.

Later in stage three he can no longer feel even partially well even if he takes his fix regularly. Without it, however, symptoms become intolerable so he is driven to take it constantly. Heavy smokers often have to have a cigarette in the middle of the night, and they certainly light up as soon as they wake in the morning. Severe hypoglycaemics have to take something to bed with them, as they often awake feeling dreadful. If it is not by their bed-side, they have to go downstairs to raid the larder or fridge.

For reasons that are not clear, the slope downwards in stage three can take years, patients only gradually going downhill. The stage at which they decide to seek medical help will depend upon a number of factors, such as the nature of the symptoms and the extent to which they are interfering with life at work and leisure.

Pure cystitis will tend only to fit into stage one, and it may stay there for a long time. On the other hand, the body could well be mainly in the early part of stage three, with other symptoms being more obviously in the addictive pattern. The cystitis may only be a sign that the body can no longer cope, and may be the result of the body desperately trying to rid itself through the kidneys of something it does not want to keep, products of allergic reactions.

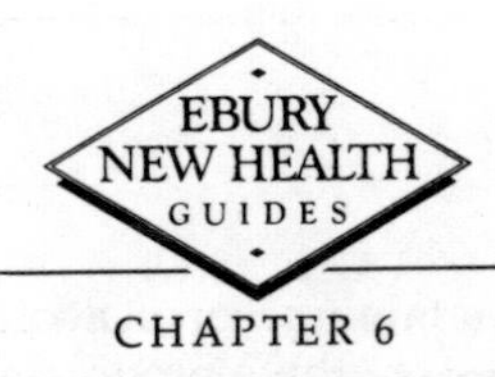

CHAPTER 6

CANDIDA

Cystitis is often the culmination of many problems, and sometimes they have accumulated over a lifetime. Frequently the main cause is the candida organism, and if this is the case its eradication is essential. The candida story is a complex one, but it is now well understood by doctors who practice clinical ecology. Its ramifications are wide and can affect any organ of the body.

Candida albicans is the mould normally responsible for thrush, a condition that tends to be associated with the female genital tract. White curd-like deposits and discharge may be found in and around the vagina; sometimes the discharge may be less copious, thick, and classically curd-like, but still cause soreness with or without itching. Very often there are symptoms of cystitis, i.e. discomfort or burning pain on passing urine, and occasionally blood in the urine. In infants, most mothers will recognize thrush as the curd-like deposits in the baby's mouth that cannot be wiped away as normal milk curds can.

Yeasts, fungi and moulds are part of nature's natural organisms, and many thousands of different species have been identified. Like the carrion crow that cleans up the countryside, moulds break down anything to its constituent parts. When food goes off, it is being attacked by a mould. When leaves rot, a mould is responsible. There is even a mould to break down concrete and others for iron and plastic, although it would take them hundreds or thousands of years to complete their task.

Moulds are an integral part of life, and they live on the skin and mucous membranes of humans. In health they cause no problems; in disease they can invade, either as the primary cause or once our defences are down. These defences are constantly eroded by what we do to ourselves, the processed food we eat, the chemicals we pollute the environment with, the drugs we take to keep ourselves going, the antibiotics we inject into animals to fatten them before slaughter.

In every patient suffering from recurrent cystitis, candida must be looked for. If it cannot be found it can be well worthwhile to treat the person as though it were present. This will do no harm at all, and in many respects it will improve the person's overall nutritional state.

Close examination of a person's secretions will reveal a mixed flora of bacteria, yeasts and moulds usually living in perfect harmony. Upset that harmony and disease sets in. Because of the continual presence of candida in and around the body, there are no standard easy tests to prove that candida is causing a problem in many people, unless there are the classical features of thrush. Then, and only then, will most doctors acknowledge that the candida organism is causing problems. Without the 'proof' the importance of candida tends to be ignored.

Over the past few years, a number of doctors, especially those who practise clinical ecology, have come to realize just how important candida can sometimes be, thanks largely to the original work of Dr. Orian Truss in the USA. Candida's importance has developed to such an extent that no self-respecting clinical ecologist dare ignore the possibility that it is a major cause of a patient's symptoms. Experience has shown that certain features in a patient's history will suggest that candida is to blame. While scientific or laboratory proof is lacking to justify candida's clinical relevance, the management and eradication of the candida mould have led to such an improvement of symptoms in so many patients that there can be little doubt left of its importance.

THE PRESENCE OF CANDIDA IN THE ABSENCE OF THRUSH

One of the main problems, however, is that orthodox medicine does not recognize that candida can be present in the absence of thrush, and even if thrush is found, it is often not considered to be a major cause of the cystitis but merely an accompaniment. All too often a patient will have recurrent episodes of candida infection, and will be given local treatment. Occasionally, an appropriate anti-fungal drug (usually nystatin) will be given by mouth, but nearly always in too small a dose and for not nearly long enough. The treatment is always in the form of a drug or medicine, with never a thought about nutrition. In fact, the nutritional approach is more effective and more long lasting. Precipitating factors must also be taken into account.

Nearly 100 per cent of the adult population has antibodies to candida in their blood, indicating that the defence mechanisms are working properly. In other words this simply means that candida has got into the tissues at some time in life and the body has set up its organization to handle each invasion. Most attacks are in the mouth or vaginal area, and the resultant thrush is a sign that the body is rejecting the candida, but that quite a battle is going on. Frequently the body needs help to win the battle.

It has been variously estimated that 90 per cent of children have candida in or on their bodies, as evidenced by the reaction to a tiny dose of candida albicans injected into the skin. This shows that the body has previously responded to the presence of candida by producing antibodies. Indeed, if a person does not show an antibody reaction to candida, it is feared there may be something wrong with their immune system. It is thought they are not able to produce antibodies in response to invasion from any pathogenic organism. The body's response to candida injection into the skin is considered a test of immune competence. Sufferers from AIDS often lack this response, and they are known to be immune deficient.

Ever since Dr. Truss put forward in the late 1970s the theory that candida was causing much ill health, there has been controversy. Clinical ecologists the world over, especially in the USA, Australia, New Zealand and the United Kingdom, accepted Dr. Truss's observations and put them to the test. The results in some patients were nothing short of astounding.

In the vast majority of my difficult patients, I have found candida to be a major contributory factor in making them feel ill, but for reasons that I could not understand until very recently, their candida seemed resistant to treatment. Despite every trick I knew, they still seemed to have candida and to be affected by it. Some of them could keep it under a degree of control, but at an expense to their life styles that was unacceptable if it continued for too long. It was plain I was missing an essential ingredient.

THE MERCURY STORY

In 1985, news came across from America that mercury leeching out of amalgam fillings in teeth was not only capable of making people ill in all sorts of ways, but was also making candida resistant to treatment. In the short time I have been dealing with the mercury problem, my hard core of difficult-to-help patients has diminished considerably. Regretfully, there will always be some I will struggle with. No doctor would ever claim to cure everyone he sees.

There has been much publicity recently about the significance of mercury in amalgam fillings, and not surprisingly the British Dental Association has denied that it is a problem. Whether they believe it or not is a matter of conjecture. Nevertheless, I am glad that they have tried to stem the tide of anxiety because we now know that it is important to confirm by various means that mercury is a problem, and it really must be dealt with in a professional way. It is vital that people should not go out and have all their amalgams removed and replaced by a suitable non-metallic substance, as the order in which this is done is absolutely vital for success and it must be done by a dentist competent and interested in this sort of work. There are many ramifications to the mercury story, which may well become as important to ill health as candida appeared to be and could well solve an enormous number of problems in some people who have, until now, resisted our best endeavours to help them get better.

NATURAL CONTROL BY THE BODY OF CANDIDA AND OTHER MOULDS

At this stage it would be useful to consider the ways the body controls candida in health, from which it will become obvious why the control breaks down.

In the healthy body, candida albicans and other moulds are present only in small numbers. They are kept under control by a number of factors which are easily destroyed by today's diet, life styles and drugs.

THE IMMUNE SYSTEM

Early on in life some candida albicans organisms penetrate into the blood stream. The body recognizes them as a foreign substance, and antibodies specific against candida albicans will be produced. In future, if the body is invaded by these organisms, those antibodies will attack and destroy them, and so prevent a candida infection. If the battle ground is a mucous membrance itself, the results will be the clinical features of thrush. So long as the body's immune system is functioning well, candida will always be kept under control.

When the environment of a particular part of the body changes to the benefit of candida, a battle is fought between the multiplying organisms and the body's immune system. If this battle ground is the warm moist vagina, which is an enclosed area, a discharge will develop as an indication that the mucous membrance has been invaded, causing the local glands to over-produce their secretions. Add to this many candida cells and the debris from their destruction, and you have the typical features of thrush – a white curd-like deposit in the vagina, vaginal discharge, and irritation and itching of the delicate area involved. Intercourse naturally becomes painful, and the woman with persistent vaginal thrush develops a fear of normal sexual relationships, often the case with a chronic cystitis sufferer.

NORMAL BOWEL FLORA

In health the bowel is colonized by millions of organisms that are friendly towards the host in which they live. The most prolific and valuable are numerous species of lactobacilli, the most common of which is *Lactobacillus acidophilus.* Even then there are various strains which are more beneficial than others, and, when supplements are given, it is helpful to choose the right one.

Early in life, *lactobacilli* colonize the bowel, along with many other organisms, some of which are potentially harmful. In the breast-fed infant, the best environment develops to encourage the implantation, growth and establishment of the most desirable organisms. Provided these grow, they outnumber all unfavourable organisms and exert a simple form of crowd control, keeping the 'baddies' in their place.

ADDITIONAL CONTROL BY LACTOBACILLI

In addition to the pure numerical advantage, *lactobacilli* produce biotin, which is part of the vitamin B complex. While the body needs a certain amount that can be obtained from food, the additional amounts produced by the presence of millions of *lactobacilli* exert a specific inhibitory influence on the yeast cells within the bowel.

OTHER EFFECTS OF THE MICROFLORA

In man and animals, surgery, drugs and other forms of stress have a profound effect upon the normal ability of the bowel to move its contents onwards. This in turn induces changes in the microflora. Some of them stimulate the muscles in the bowel wall to make it function normally, and normal bowel function helps keep the microflora normal. Disturb either and both are affected.

The normal friendly organisms can stop candida and other potentially harmful organisms from sticking to the mucosa of the bowel. If the candida cells cannot actually reach the bowel wall they cannot invade the tissues. By being kept away from the wall itself, the unwanted cells can be more easily excreted.

SHORT CHAIN FATTY-ACIDS

A healthy diet produces short chain fatty-acids during the process of the digestion of food. These substances are also produced by *lactobacilli* and other friendly organisms that inhabit the normal bowel. Laboratory experiments have demonstrated that some of these chemicals, notably caprylic acid, help keep candida albicans under control.

THE EFFECT OF FIBRE

It is well known that a high fibre diet improves constipation, by increasing the activity of the muscles in the bowel wall. Normal bowel action is influenced by the amount of fibre inside it. If the diet is low in fibre, there is little for the bowel wall to work on, and so constipation occurs leading to stagnation of its contents.

When the contents of the bowel move slowly through its interior, potentially pathogenic bacteria have an opportunity to develop and become established. When there is plenty of fibre which is not absorbed but passes through the whole length of the bowel, organisms are trapped within its meshes and so prevented from contacting the bowel wall and becoming established. The more the natural fibre content of the food up to a certain extent, the more active the bowel becomes, the more it cleanses the bowel of potentially harmful organisms, and the more a normal microflora becomes established. For these and many other reasons a healthy diet has obvious benefits.

FEATURES IN A PATIENT'S PAST HISTORY THAT ARE LINKED TO CANDIDA

There is no doubt whatsoever that antibiotics have saved countless thousands of lives since their introduction into medicine in the 1940s, prior to which people died far too easily from infections, or had intractable long-term consequences of that infection such as osteomyelitis. Nevertheless, their use has been abused, and they have been given far too often when they were not indicated, or when simple alternative measures would have been just as effective. Antibiotics should only be given when they are needed.

Frequent Courses of Antibiotics

Going into a person's medical history by asking specific questions, I frequently find that in their childhood they suffered from tonsillitis, ear problems, bronchitis, more coughs and colds than usual, or from any condition that was called an infection. Not surprisingly, an antibiotic was given with the result that, as a child, the patient had many courses of antibiotics each year for a number of years.

All too frequently these episodes that kept recurring, just like recurrent cystitis, were not really infections but were in fact allergic reactions to something in their diet, most commonly cow's milk. Once the area involved – for example the tonsils – became inflamed by the allergic reaction, it would clearly become an ideal breeding ground for germs which would not only continue the condition but make it worse. Thus, the tonsils would eventually become infected and an antibiotic called for. I am not arguing that antibiotics should not have been given at all, but once a couple of attacks had occurred, someone should have asked the question why.

Acne

Teenagers often suffer from acne at a time when they are trying to develop socially, and when a spotty face is a great drawback. One of the standard treatments is a broad spectrum antibiotic called tetracycline, often given for months or years to control the germs that grow in the skin. Some antibiotics such as penicillin, are fairly narrow in the range of pathogenic bacteria they kill. Ampicillin, tetracycline and others, especially the ones that are poorly absorbed from the gastro-intestinal tract such as neomycin, have such a wide spectrum of activity against organisms that they kill virtually everything in their way, including the harmless organisms needed by the gut.

Having destroyed the organisms useful to your intestines, candida is left free to grow unopposed. As an opportunist organism, candida will multiply and the rate at which it grows will depend upon many things, such as the environment within the intestines. If there is a high intake of refined carbohydrate and very little roughage, candida will grow well. If there is high roughage and low carbohydrate, candida may struggle, and the re-growth of the valuable organisms may restart and soon bring the imbalance back to normal again.

The effect of a single course of a broad spectrum antibiotic on the intestinal flora of a nutritionally sound person may be minimal, but a nutritionally-neglected person who is given frequent courses of antibiotics will soon become affected by candida. If candida is not considered as a cause of the continuing ill-health, the patient may well fail to recover.

Problems of Female Reproductive Organs

I am now firmly convinced that candida can produce a number of problems, in fact probably almost any problem associated with the female reproductive organs. Many women tell me that their periods were painful and heavy from the minute they started. A lot of these women were given antibiotics in childhood for the reasons already described, and so candida could well have started invading the womb and ovaries before puberty. Some of these women are so badly affected they end up having a hysterectomy. Although this temporarily 'cures' the problem because the target organ for the symptoms has been removed from the body, ill health invariably occurs months or even years later.

Of course, many women are told that their periods will improve after pregnancy. To be fair they often do. However, there can be a few days of severe pain and debility every month for many years from the onset of periods aged eleven or twelve to the time of the first pregnancy. It is possible that the stretching of the muscles of the womb by the growing baby has an effect like stretching a leg muscle that has gone into cramp. Alternatively, there is a lot of extra zinc in the womb of a pregnant woman which may locally help the immune system repel candida.

Some women who had painful periods before their pregnancies have painful periods afterwards. Fortunately, they are a minority, but they tend to be the ones who end up having a hysterectomy. They will also be more likely to have had some sort of difficulty with one or more of their births, either an early or late one, or a comparatively complicated one, which is suggestive of a zinc deficiency. They are therefore less inclined to risk another awkward birth and are more likely to be willing to submit to a hysterectomy.

If a young girl complains of too painful periods, it is quite likely she will be put onto the pill for therapeutic reasons and, since ovulation is prevented by the pill, subsequent periods are likely to be far shorter in duration and possibly virtually painless. So, while the pill can help the symptoms of painful periods, it may actually make the whole picture worse by further encouraging the candida which may have been the cause in the first place.

A common symptom in women affected by candida is the premenstrual syndrome; however there are other causes of it. Some women with candida suffer both premenstrual symptoms and painful periods, and in these patients the control of candida may well bring immeasurable relief. While the symptoms of abdominal bloating, breast tenderness, fluid accumulation, migraines, irritability or depression may occur for a few days before the onset of a period, some women suffer two weeks in every month from premenstrual symptoms, plus one week of the period itself. Quite commonly, food allergies appear in the premenstrual times only to disappear at the onset of the period.

The Contraceptive Pill

As a contraceptive, the pill clearly has many advantages. But despite soothing words of comfort from various authorities there is disquiet amongst many doctors and health professionals about its safety.

There is little doubt, for instance, that the pill brings an increased risk of developing thrush. Many women on the pill have an increased vaginal discharge which defies explanation. In a percentage of them, it is candida without the usual clinical manifestations of thrush. When the pill is stopped the discharge often improves, but it may well not, suggesting that the pill has induced a state of candidosis which does not go away on stopping the pill, unless other anti-candida measures are taken.

Despite a history of problems at various stages of life suggesting that candida may have been involved, many women say they have never been well since starting the contraceptive pill, or 'since the children were born'. The taking of a tablet containing a small amount of oestrogen and progesterone is similar to the state of pregnancy, in which it is firmly established that vaginal thrush can develop. It seems likely therefore that the pill is a precipitating factor in the development of candidosis in many women.

The pill can unbalance the intestinal flora. On its own this may not lead to frank candidosis, but when other factors are present like a couple of courses of broad-spectrum antibiotics too close together, plus a diet too high in refined carbohydrates, the pill may be the last straw. It may only need one or two months on the pill to set things going.

Apart from its candida-promoting effects, the pill leads to deficiencies of a number of essential nutrients, especially zinc, vitamin C, vitamin B6 and other B vitamins. This makes the immune system less efficient, rendering the body less capable of resisting invasion by candida. On its own, then, the contraceptive pill can have two independent effects, the first candida-promoting, the second leading to deficiencies of certain essential nutrients. Unfortunately, the two together tend to have a multiplying rather than an additive effect, while each one individually can help the development of food and chemical allergies.

Hormone replacement therapy

After the menopause, many women develop a dryness of the vagina and other symptoms such as suddenly appearing older than their natural age, or brittle bones. This suggests to many doctors that the person is suffering from a loss of female hormones, mainly oestrogen. While that may well be the effect, the cause is often food allergies supressing the natural output or causing their sudden demise.

In a healthy woman before the menopause there are day-to-day and hour-to-hour variations in the amount of oestrogen put out, largely by the ovaries but also to a small extent by the adrenal glands. Around the menopause, the output by the ovaries gradually wanes, also with day-to-day variations. Eventually it virtually stops, although a small amount is usually produced for many years. Provided the change has taken place normally and smoothly, and the person was fit and well before the onset of the change, the post-menopausal phase should proceed without any problems at all.

Many women who suffer around the time of the menopause, and who are put onto hormone replacement therapy, were also unwell before the change of life. If their problems had been sorted out before the menopause, the need for hormone replacement therapy could well have been avoided. Once the condition has arisen, it is difficult to make a person feel well without continuing to use these hormones.

Unfortunately, because hormone replacement therapy is an oestrogen, and taking a pill does not vary the blood levels in the way it occurs in the natural state, the development of candida is encouraged.

Corticosteroids

Corticosteroids such as prednisolone and ACTH (adrenocorticotrophic hormone) are commonly used in a number of medical conditions such as asthma, colitis and arthritis, although most doctors try to avoid their use.

To achieve their effect in these medical conditions, corticosteroids suppress inflammatory reactions. This may be desirable when inflammation is causing unacceptable symptoms that cannot be adequately controlled in any other way, or when the patient's very life is threatened as in severe asthma. These chemical drugs suppress all inflammation, which is the body's normal response to any invader, be it a splinter or a pathogenic bacterium. Thus the body's ability to fight an invasion of candida or any unfriendly organism is compromised. Many patients on corticosteroids are also given regular antibiotics for this very reason.

Another unfortunate problem with corticosteroids is that they produce a diabetes-like condition, and indeed frank diabetes can develop. These steroids cause an increase in the total amount of sugar in the person thus providing a readily available source of food for candida organisms. Their development is therefore guaranteed. When a person has been on corticosteroids for a long period of time, the body's ability to produce its own cortisol becomes affected. This makes it all the more difficult to get the patient off steroids, making the eradication of candida that much more difficult.

Tablets of corticosteroids and injections of ACTH are used by doctors as seldom as possible but inhalers for use in the nose and lungs are frequently prescribed for rhinitis (blockage and running of the nose) and asthma.

Many studies have confirmed that these inhaled steroids promote the growth of candida, and those used for asthma often cause hoarseness and a sore throat because of the presence of the unwanted organism. Anti-candida gargles may be used, but, by and large, the patient is told to put up with it because the inhaled steroids are controlling his asthma and making the oral form, with all its attendant problems, unnecessary.

Frequently, of course, the presence of candida goes unnoticed or unlooked for. On the assumption that it develops in the throat, it can gradually pass the whole length of the intestines and start to cause other symptoms. It would certainly help if the anti-candida diet was started, in which case candida might not develop in the first place, and its spread would probably be avoided.

Pregnancy

Orthodox medicine knows that candida in the vagina commonly occurs during pregnancy. There is more sugar around the uterus in order to sustain the fetus, and the mucus in the vagina changes to make the environment more suitable for candida to develop.

Sickness in pregnancy is often the result of poor diet, or zinc or magnesium deficiencies, and once it has occurred it is hardly likely to encourage a woman to eat properly. She is therefore all the more likely to eat what she fancies, i.e. sugary things and cups of tea or coffee;

certainly not the foods that might help correct any nutritional deficiencies she is already suffering from.

Thus candida can develop and proliferate, remembering that it is a normal inhabitant of the vagina and the skin between the legs, but that its growth is inhibited by the correct environment. In pregnancy that environment changes to one more conducive to its development.

Many women notice how their health has deteriorated with each pregnancy, and the more children someone has, the greater the problem each time. If she becomes pregnant soon after stopping breast feeding the previous child, her chances of recovering to a state fit enough to feed the next child will be all the less. The more children she has, the smaller is likely to be the gap between each, and the greater the problem for her. Often, however, women with large families feed themselves and their family well, not allowing sweets and junk food into the house.

The comparison between the state of pregnancy and taking the contraceptive pill is an interesting one. The nutritional status of a woman who is on the pill for ten years might be quite similar to one who has had six children in ten years, and breast fed each one for between six and nine months.

Thrush

Regular episodes of thrush are clearly an indication of challenge by candida, a challenge in which the candida appears to be winning. Usually treatment is given in the form of nystatin or a similar topically-applied anti-fungal antibiotic, which helps the body to win the battle. Unfortunately, regular episodes of thrush are nearly always treated with another course of the same or an alternative drug, again applied to the local area in the form of vaginal pessaries and creams, and occasionally a short course, say one week, of oral nystatin. While this might help, it seldom goes far enough and attention is rarely paid to the diet, a change of which can be so beneficial.

Many women with recurrent cystitis find a close association with thrush, but I often find that thrush has been something they used to suffer from and in fact don't suffer from so badly now. In fact they often feel that their cystitis has got worse since their thrush stopped troubling them, although the occasional attack can still occur, normally in a milder form. It is as if they have swapped thrush for cystitis. For want of a better explanation, it is as if the candida organism has turned inwards, and is no longer attacking the local tissues round the vagina and urethra. It has presumably changed from its yeast form to the mycelial form, and has invaded deeper. In these circumstances thrush symptoms are absent and so the possibility that candida is causing the problem is never seriously thought of. A urine sample will in fact seldom show candida to be present, as it is no longer on the surface to contaminate the urine.

CLINICAL FEATURES THAT SUGGEST CANDIDA MAY BE INVOLVED

As a result of good clinical observations, doctors practising clinical ecology have come to realize that many symptoms that patients regularly complain of and which are treated by all sorts of drugs, very often without success, can be caused by candida. That is not to say that whenever a patient complains of any of the symptoms listed below, candida is always the cause. Many food reactions can produce the same symptoms. Take coffee as an example. In one person it can cause headaches, in another pain around the heart, in a third palpitations, while in others it can cause arthritis, backache, sleeplessness, anxiety, depression, fatigue, inability to cope, all as individual symptoms or as a mixture of any of them. One just needs to be aware that the problems candida can cause in anyone are many and varied. Having said that, there are certain features that seem to occur when candida is involved.

Mental Symptoms

These can be very variable, but those most commonly found in patients affected by candida are mental confusion, inability to concentrate, forgetfulness, mental fatigue, depression and mood swings. While the classical diagnoses of manic depression, schizophrenia, and severe depression may involve candida, there are usually important causes such as lead intoxication, zinc deficiency, milk, wheat or coffee allergies. Each must be looked for.

Skin Problems

Virtually any skin complaint can be caused by, or certainly exacerbated by candida. The common skin problems most closely associated with candida, however, are chronic urticaria (hives), psoriasis, and any fungal infection, for example athlete's foot, and fungal infections between the buttocks and in the groin. Fungal infections of the toenails are not uncommon, if looked for, but they are seldom seen on fingernails, although what may be considered as eczema between the fingers can often be a fungal infection. A particularly nasty form of arthritis involving the finger and toenails is called psoriatic arthritis. In many ways it is very similar to rheumatoid arthritis, but it has the peculiar involvement of the nails. In such a condition the treatment of choice must centre around candida.

While the relationship between candida and psoriasis has only been acknowledged by clinical ecologists in the past handful of years, homoeopathy made an interesting connection between the two nearly 200 years ago. One of the standard and very successful homoeopathic treatments for female thrush is borax. When I looked up borax in the homoeopathic *Materia Medica,* I found it was also definitely indicated in the management of psoriasis.

Abdominal Symptoms

Since the candida organism tends to pool in the intestine, probably the large intestine, it is not surprising that intestinal symptoms of any sort may be connected with the candida problem. Abdominal pain, constipation, diarrhoea, bloating, wind both up and down, a foul taste in the mouth, and 'rumblings', can all occur, although strangely some people with definite candida may not have any significant symptoms coming from the intestinal tract at all.

Whatever the involvement, treatment of candida usually leads to a change in bowel function. If constipation, diarrhoea or wind were the main features, these usually improve quite rapidly. On the other hand, if the bowel were considered comparatively normal before treatment, increased activity not uncommonly occurs, but usually not for long as the bowel eliminates the candida organisms.

It must be remembered that any drug, medicine or nutritional supplements may be capable of having a side-effect in an individual patient. The various forms used in the treatment of candida, while acceptable to most patients, are also capable of producing undesirable side-effects. Sometimes the treatment has to be stopped, although if it is restarted at a different dose the effect may not recur.

Problems of the Female Reproductive Organs

In patients with recurrent cystitis, there may be concurrent problems of premenstrual tension, heavy and painful periods and pain at ovulation. Sometimes PMT begins at ovulation, giving a woman only one reasonable week in every four – not a very pleasant way of living, especially if attacks of cystitis crop up now and then.

The reason why I have already discussed this problem in the previous section is because frequently these symptoms occurred some time in the past, but are no longer of major importance. It is almost as though the body tried to draw attention to something being wrong only for it to be ignored (by being treated with a drug instead of finding out the cause and dealing with it). These symptoms often occur before the first pregnancy, i.e. throughout the teens and early twenties, only to be 'interrupted' by starting a family. On occasions the original symptoms recur between each pregnancy, or start again after a suitable interval, say two to three years, after the last baby is born.

Again, it is almost as if the body is putting off telling you about something being wrong, while it concentrates on trying to bring a new off-spring successfully into the world. Often, of course, it has difficulty in achieving this. After a child is born symptoms may not recur for two to three years, almost as if the body is waiting for the woman to make up her mind whether to get pregnant again or not.

Candida and Men: Prostatism

While most problems with candida affect women, it must not be forgotten that men can be affected. Doctors seldom think men can have candida because they seldom see thrush in an adult male, unless he has 'caught it' from his female partner, and even then it is likely only to be found on his penis. So any evidence of prostatism should raise the question of candida.

Symptoms are a difficulty in starting to pass urine and an inadequate end, often dribbling being a nuisance. The amount passed at any one time may be small, and there may soon be a need to go again. An examination by a doctor will reveal an enlarged prostate. The usual treatment is its removal (a prostatectomy), but it leads to impotency in far too many men. In general, however, it tends to be a condition of older men who may not be concerned with such a side-effect of the operation. In younger men, it can obviously be a great disadvantage.

While men don't take the pill or have replacement hormones, they can, of course, be given corticosteroids for ulcerative colitis, asthma, etc. On the other hand, they are just as likely as women to have been given antibiotics in childhood, and indeed young men from puberty into their twenties often suffer from acne, for which one standard treatment is daily antibiotics, often for years. Thus candida must not be forgotten as a possible cause of problems in the male.

Craving

As candida feeds on sugar, many patients crave sweets, sugar, foods with sugar such as chocolate, cream buns, etc, and white flour products such as white bread. The symptoms are headaches, mental confusion, lightheadedness, fatigue, palpitations, a gnawing feeling in the pit of the stomach, sweating and pins and needles.

On occasions, patients crave yeast-containing foods and beverages such as cheese, yeast extracts and alcohol. Bread is a common food to crave and of course, it contains yeast and refined carbohydrate if it is white bread. Many people simply 'like' cheese, so it is sometimes difficult to separate a 'liking' from a 'craving'. There are times, however, when a patient says 'I couldn't do without cheese!' On that evidence it probably must be avoided.

As with most symptoms, the cravings settle well when candida is brought under control. However, when the craving is considerable – and it is sometimes overwhelming – it can require immense effort to stop eating that particular food. So it is only sensible to make sure that the foods craved are completely removed from the house.

Generally Feeling Unwell

This really is a rag-bag of problems, so much so that doctors nearly always recommend psychiatric referral. Yet many sufferers from candida just don't feel very well, and there seems to be no good reason for their symptoms. They may feel lethargic, a bit headachy, ache a little, feel as if they can't be bothered, a touch anxious, don't sleep too well, yet mope about much of the day feeling tired and run down.

Complaints of this sort to their doctor may well result in a batch of blood tests, X-rays, urine tests, possibly an examination of thyroid function, but usually nothing will be found to be wrong, so a diagnosis of endogenous depression or something psychosomatic will be made and an anti-depressant or tranquillizer tried, sometimes making the patient feel even more like a zombie than before.

If the brain and body are being affected by candida and food allergies so that the chemical mechanisms are being disturbed, it doesn't really make sense to add a drug which is also capable of affecting the chemicals in the brain. It is not surprising, therefore, that many people who are put onto these drugs actually feel worse. In my mind such an observation is tantamount to saying the person *does* have a food or chemical allergy or a candida problem.

Mouldy Conditions

Some patients with candida feel their symptoms more on damp days and in mouldy places. Candida can be stimulated to activity by a cross-reaction with other moulds and yeasts, which is why the treatment involves eliminating all yeast-type foods from the diet. Potted plants harbour moulds, especially in the soil in the base of the pot, so they should be removed from the house. If they are special favourites, lend them to a relative or friend, preferably whose house you are not likely to visit too often. With any luck you will be able to have them back before too long. Try to avoid visiting places with lots of potted plants.

Check your own house for moulds. The easiest places to miss are clothes cupboards (especially built-in ones), and in particular any on outside walls. As the doors are kept closed most of the time, air does not circulate properly except when you open them to get something out or put something in. Remember, you spend one third of your lifetime in bed in the bedroom, so you could be constantly exposed to an unnecessary amount of mould spores in the air you breathe in every night.

Other places to have checked (preferably by someone else) are the cupboard under the kitchen sink, and behind and under the bottom shelf of bookshelves, especially if they touch the floor. Also have the downstairs toilet and cupboard under the stairs checked. The area of the house most likely to be mouldy is downstairs because it is closest to the dampness of the soil around the house, and any closed area should be thoroughly inspected. A cellar is a very likely place for moulds to grow, and spores from down there can invade the air of the ground floor. Check this out thoroughly.

Many candida sufferers fail to understand why they feel so unwell after working in the garden, especially in autumn. The answer should be perfectly plain by now – they disturb mould working on the soil, breaking down leaves, etc. Compost heaps and raking leaves can be particularly bad, and gardening should be avoided if at all possible.

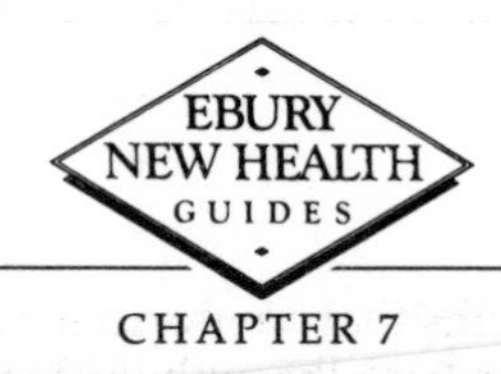

CHAPTER 7

TAKING THE PATIENT'S HISTORY

In Chapter Four, I explained my concept of ill health and showed how it differs from the views currently accepted by the majority of doctors. The orthodox attitude is that the organ that is producing symptoms should be the focus of attention, and the whole of the treatment should concentrate on that organ. The orthodox approach is to treat the patient with drugs and see if he or she improves. If that doesn't work, then the answer may well be in surgery.

My attitude is completely different. I believe that the body has natural inbuilt mechanisms for normality, and that the body prefers to be normal if it is given a chance. If you can find out what is upsetting the body and you remove it, the body will recover and return to normal, and the symptoms will disappear. If the body has given a warning by producing some sort of symptom which is ignored or suppressed by a drug, that problem will come out in another way later on, remembering that the body is capable of 'adapting'. Thus I believe that if you do not find out the *cause* of some minor trouble that occurs at any time in life, then, as the cause has not been dealt with (even if the symptoms have), that same cause will most likely surface elsewhere at another time.

If you put a stone on a weed, you temporarily hide it from view. In due course, however, it will grow round the edge and appear once again, sometimes stronger than before. If, instead of putting a stone on it, you cut the weed off just below the surface of the soil so that it is no longer visible, it will eventually grow again, this time thicker and stronger. If it is dug out by the roots, the problem will be solved and that weed will not appear again.

The situation is very similar in man. Get to the root cause of the problem and deal with it properly, and the matter is at an end. Do a partial job and, while the matter may temporarily appear to have been dealt with, it will come back with a vengeance. In human disease terms, this means finding out 'why'.

The patient's history is important to me because it means I can trace back the various problems that have arisen over a lifetime. In fact it is quite reasonable to trace back through the family, as there is plenty of evidence to suggest that an allergic parent will have an allergic child. Treat the parent before conception and the chances of a normal child are greatly improved.

By going back into the history, I hope to explain why problems have arisen, what their causes are, and how they could have been dealt with had the patient been seen by a doctor with my medical attitude. While the person's clock cannot be turned back to pretend that the problem has never existed, obtaining a detailed history and explaining what it means gives the patient confidence that the approach I am about to suggest will be worth following.

Despite the many problems a patient may have had in the past, I am amazed at the body's remarkable potential for recovery. Severe symptoms that have lasted for many years can often completely disappear leaving no trace of their previous existence.

It has to be appreciated, however, that some conditions do leave their mark. The person whose diabetes has led to the amputation of a leg cannot have that leg back. A patient with severe recurrent cystitis who has had an 'operation' of some sort, possibly fashioning a new bladder or making the opening to the outside somewhere else instead of the normal channel through the urethra, cannot go back to square one. The person who has had part of his stomach removed because of an ulcer cannot have that part returned to him.

To be able to help someone get better, I have to ask all the right questions and make sure I understand exactly what the patient means. Many years ago, I asked a woman if she opened her bowels regularly, to which she replied 'Yes, thank you.' I later asked her how often she opened her bowels, to which she replied 'Regularly once every two weeks!' Both answers were correct but the second far more informative!

At the beginning of my meeting with a new patient, I explain my philosophy of how illnesses come about. At various times I tell stories about other patients (not naming them of course), showing how I tracked down that patient's problems, even if it took rather a lot of digging. Sometimes it was easy. Often the patients actually knew what the cause was but ignored the signs. My prompting made them realize how simple it was.

About a year ago, a girl in her late teens (I shall call her Jenny) was brought to see me by her parents. She was complaining of constipation, abdominal pain and bloating of her tummy. She had been through the usual medical investigations and the final offer was for a surgeon to open her up and 'have a look inside'. In answer to her parents' questions, the specialist had said that he didn't think he would find anything wrong but would do the operation 'just in case'.

Part of my history-taking includes asking if the patient is aware that any foods upset her. Often a person knows that onions and cucumber, for example, cause indigestion, but a patient often avoids certain foods because she knows they upset her. In answer to my question, Jenny said that oranges made her lips swell.

I began to write down 'Avoids oranges as they make her lips swell', saying it out loud as I did so. Before I had completed the sentence, Jenny said 'No, I don't avoid them'. It turned out that, since she loved oranges so much but they had this unfortunate effect if they simply touched her lips, she had found that she could continue to enjoy them so long as she parted her lips with the fingers of her left hand as she popped the orange segments in with her other hand! It had never occurred to her or her parents that her bloated tummy was caused by the oranges. She had ignored the warning signs and had found a way round them to her peril. On avoiding oranges altogether all her tummy problems went away. On eating oranges again, they came back. This is one of my standard stories, but there are others. They help the patient get onto my wave length, and to think of things that might be worth mentioning to me as possible causes of their symptoms. I never mind how bizarre or comical they might be. I encourage the patient to suggest anything. If I think it a possibility, we can always put it to the test somehow. I want the patient to share ideas with me.

In the process of obtaining a detailed history, I am given the opportunity not only to get to know the patient, but also to dig out the important aspects of their life so far. When trying to find out why a patient recently had an apparently high level of lead in his body which could possibly contribute to his arthritis, he explained how for more than forty years, in fact since the age of six, he had pinched lead weights onto the end of his fishing line with his teeth, until his arthritis had stopped him from enjoying his hobby a number of years ago. I felt satisfied I had uncovered the source of lead in his body.

MY APPROACH TO TAKING A CASE HISTORY

The orthodox medical approach is to deal with the situation as it applies now. I go back into the patient's history and try to trace as many events as possible. This makes me (and the patient) open the net as wide as possible, and makes us both consider the most insignificant event that might explain something. A patient who complained of conjunctivitis (an irritation in the eyes) went to stay with an old school friend for a week during which time her symptoms disappeared entirely, only to return when she got home. It turned out it was the pink and blue dyes in the tissues she used to cleanse her face in the morning and evening that were causing her problems. When she stayed with her friend she used the white tissues her friend provided. Her lucky break away from home gave me the clue. Had it not occurred at that particular time, I could so easily have missed the chance to help her. Following that experience I have discovered that the colours used in toilet paper can be a major cause of cystitis in some patients.

THE HISTORY IN THE FIRST FEW YEARS OF LIFE

If the patient in front of me is an adult, especially an elderly person, they may have no knowledge of their mother's condition near the time she conceived the patient or delivered her. If a woman is accompanied by the mother, the picture is often fascinating.

Frequently the mother was on the contraceptive pill for a number of years, coming off it 'to start a family'. The pill causes loss of certain vitamins and minerals so that the mother may have achieved a pregnancy being somewhat deficient in some of them. Frequently these deficiencies, especially that of zinc, can lead to a difficulty in conceiving. The child is therefore born with its health somewhat compromised and has a greater chance of developing allergies.

In fact, the first sign of allergies may be an unduly active or quiet baby in the womb. The active child may well turn so many times that he has the cord twisted round his neck at birth. Once born, the baby may appear 'unsatisfied' by its mother's milk, despite her appearing to produce enough. Usually, if she stops taking cow's milk products herself, her milk 'improves', and the baby's symptoms subside. How can her baby say that there is something in its mother's breast milk that is upsetting it, without crying. That is all the baby can do, usually with abdominal colic as well. More snuffles than usual, any infection in the ears, throat and chest, or eczema, all point to a cow's milk allergy, although other foods can be implicated. An orthodox doctor will treat the regular 'infections' with antibiotics, thereby upsetting the intestinal flora and predisposing the patient to candida and other moulds.

THE HISTORY DURING THE SCHOOL YEARS

I am not aware there is any major significance in whether a child does or does not develop the usual childhood illnesses such as chickenpox or measles, although a nutritionally deficient child may well succumb more easily, and may possibly be more seriously affected and take longer to recover. Certainly these diseases can devastate the young in the areas of the world where serious malnourishment is a real problem. Their immune system is known to be most inefficient.

Many of my patients had their tonsils and adenoids removed. As they are the first lymph glands of the body to be exposed to inhaled germs, they are constantly repelling the invaders and tend to swell from constant use. Add to this the 'infections' regularly suffered by many children that are really the lymph glands responding to an allergic reaction, and it is easy to see why they eventually become very enlarged.

Although the operation to remove the tonsils and adenoids was in vogue throughout the forties and fifties, tonsillitis and adenitis of sufficient frequency and severity to lead to their removal is always a strong indication of many allergic reactions in the past, most commonly to cow's milk.

Hyperactivity, poor attention span, failure to progress at school as well as expected, are all signs of a reaction to something being eaten or drunk. Behavioural problems, headaches, unreasonable hunger, undue thirst (often for orange squash containing tartrazine E102), weight gain, a dishevelled appearance, acne and bad skin, dark rings under the eyes (called allergic shiners), unreasonable rejection of parents' advice and concern, teenage moodiness, growing pains, etc., are such common events nowadays that they are considered 'part of growing up'. I do not agree. They are signs that something is wrong, and it is important that the cause be detected and dealt with.

I always ask when a girl's periods began and what they were like. Undue problems such as premenstrual tension (with depression, bloating, backache and pins and needles a few days before the onset of periods etc.) are frequently acknowledged. The period is often painful and flows for seven days with clots in the first day or two. The patient may well have had to go to bed for one or two days every month. This suggests congestion in the womb caused by food allergies or candida. Again, the food most commonly implicated is cow's milk.

Unfortunately, many girls who suffer from painful periods or from premenstrual tension are put onto the contraceptive pill. As this prevents ovulation, the cycle is considerably altered and the effect is to reduce the congestion and pain of the period and the premenstrual build up. While this can temporarily have a most beneficial affect, it builds up a problem for the future, in particular causing a deficiency of certain vitamins and minerals such as vitamin B6, zinc and magnesium, as well as making the development of candida all the more likely.

If a woman has been on the pill for some years and then stops it to try to start a family and succeeds in getting pregnant straightaway, she will lose more nutrients to her developing baby from her already depleted body. At worst, she may not be able to supply enough nutrition to her baby, which may either develop a congenital malformation such as spina bifida or a hare-lip, or be born prematurely, for example. The mother herself will suffer by being left with insufficient nutrients for herself. During pregnancy her altered hormone levels are likely to protect her, and she may remain remarkably well while breast feeding. A few week after weaning, however, she may start feeling unwell.

In fact, a failure to conceive, or an early miscarriage can be caused by nutrient deficiencies (notably zinc), by candida or by food allergies. Unreasonable nausea in the early stages of the pregnancy is often a sign of a zinc or magnesium deficiency or an unsuitable diet. Some women can feel sick throughout the whole nine months. An early or late delivery (provided the obstetrician has not interfered) with or without problems during labour strongly suggests a zinc deficiency. Some women struggle to produce a smallish baby, say 6 lb to $6^1/_2$ lb, without there being any structural reason to explain it. Other women manage to deliver an 8 lb to 9 lb baby without any difficulty.

All of these features in the history suggest reasons why the body has failed to cope over the past years, and why the patient is now ill and seeking medical help. Had she been seen by a clinical ecologist or a nutritional physician in the past, simple measures could have been instituted and future problems prevented.

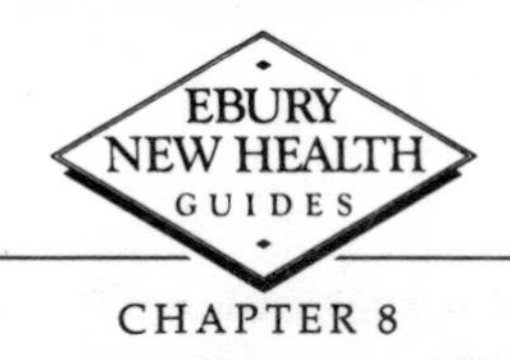

CHAPTER 8

A TYPICAL CASE HISTORY

SOME patients become ill for no reason that they can explain, yet precipitating and predisposing factors can usually be unearthed for the history. At the first interview, patients may be alone, although I always encourage them to be accompanied by a close relative or friend, in front of whom they do not mind exposing their personal medical history. What they do not know or cannot remember from my questions they can think about later and answer when I see them the next time.

Because a full medical and family history can be so revealing, it is worth describing a typical patient. I am sure many of you reading this story will recognize yourselves, and feel that certain parts of it are similar to your own history.

ANN WATSON

When I first saw her, Ann Watson was 33 years old, five feet four inches tall, and somewhat overweight at $10^1/_2$ st (147 lb or 66.8 kg). She was married with a son aged nine and a daughter aged six. Her husband, Ken, was a hard-working man of thirty-five, who just could not understand what was wrong with her. He came with her each time because he loved her and wanted to help in any way he could.

Ann's Problems: When asked, Ann said her problems had started about three years ago when she began having crying spells, low moods and no real interest in life. Ken, in turn, said these episodes of depression (Ann did not like his using this word) seemed to come out of the blue, and she herself could not explain them. After all, she had a happy marriage, a loving, caring and hard-working husband, their own house in a nice area, and two lovely children. Ann's parents lived eight miles away so she saw them regularly, although Ken's were 80 miles away and they did not see so much of them. Ken had been promoted to

District Sales Manager a year ago, so they really did not have any money problems.

A clear history of symptoms coming out of the blue is typical of food allergies. If symptoms come on a short time after eating a normal meal or having a cup of tea or coffee, and the patient is reacting to one or more items just taken, symptoms will be described as 'coming out of the blue', if the connection is not made. It is obvious if you develop a rash after eating strawberries on the odd occasion in the summer, or are sick after eating shellfish while on holiday.

Further details: Ann gradually elaborated and explained that her 'attacks', as she called them, could come on at any time of the day, even at weekends when Ken was at home. They did not happen every day by any means, but could occur three or four times a week, lasting for about 20 minutes to half a day, although sometimes much longer. Once she had felt miserable for two days after the wedding of a close friend. She and Ken had intended to make an evening of it with some friends they had met that afternoon, but, just as most of the other guests started going home, Ann had begun to feel unwell, headachey and exhausted. By the time she had got to the car for Ken to drive her home, she was in floods of tears, and Ken got cross with her for the first time. Obviously she had spoiled what should have been a fun day, especially as her mother was having the kids to stay overnight and they only had themselves to think of for a change.

If you are allergic to a food you are eating regularly, the symptoms will be masked. When you stop eating that food, the allergy is unmasked and withdrawal symptoms develop. To complicate the picture, a person may start to develop symptoms as a result of eating a food to which she is becoming allergic. Except in the obvious situation of an allergy to strawberries, for example, it is unusual for a patient to be sensitive to only one food. The more foods the patient is sensitive to, the more complicated the picture.

In fact Ann could not understand it herself. She had been looking forward to her friend's wedding. The weather had been glorious, and she had met three friends from school, and they had thoroughly enjoyed hearing all their news. The buffet meal was excellent and she had not had too much to drink, so it did not make any sense to her at all.

The clue here is the buffet meal. For a week or so Ann may have gone on a diet to look good at the wedding of her friend, or to be able to fit more easily into a particular outfit. Then, at the wedding itself, she probably ate some white bread sandwiches and had some cake and other things to which she started reacting. Having probably avoided them for a number of days before the wedding, she was now in a heightened state of sensitivity, and soon started to suffer. Add to that some alcohol, and a severe 'reaction' was inevitable. Alcohol always potentiates (make worse) any allergic reaction.

The story unravels: As usual, she got over the attack, but she felt pretty low for the next two days. That evening she went to bed early, and got up at 10.00 am the next morning after 13 hours sleep, feeling a little hung-over. A couple of cups of strong black coffee helped her a little, but she was by no means feeling well when she and Ken went over to her parents for lunch and to pick up the kids. The attack seemed so pointless and unexplainable, but it had left a firm impression in her memory. She and Ken had gone over it a number of times since, trying to sort it all out. Her general practitioner, who had been very kind, could not explain it either. It went down as 'just one of those things'.

Reactions can last many days, although they often last only a few hours. It is not surprising Ann felt bad for a few days after so bad a reaction. She could have felt better if she had taken a mixture of sodium bicarbonate and Epsom Salts (or potassium bicarbonate) in water. The pick-me-up effect of strong, black coffee has been known for years, and it can often have this effect, whatever the cause of the low mood. It is particularly effective if the depression is a withdrawal symptom from the previous cup of coffee. However, once this effect has worn off, the original symptoms will come back again.

The next two years: However, similar episodes appeared from time to time, each one with its own variations, but always the same sort of pattern. Some lasted longer, some shorter. What was particularly frightening, however, was the insidious change that took place over the next two years. Although the attacks were never as bad as the particular one on her friend's wedding day, the episodes began to last longer and longer. What was all the more alarming to Ken was that she did not really clear completely in between. She seemed permanently a little low, miserable, lethargic, lacking in interest and tired. They stopped going out to parties and dinner with friends, and certainly Ann could not be bothered to cook and entertain their friends. It had all become too much trouble.

Patients with a typical allergy like hay fever will often tell you that their attacks are not always at their worst when the pollen count is at its highest. The humidity, wind and other factors seem to affect them. With Ann, she no doubt ate more bread on some days than others. When food reactions first occur, they are often quite dramatic, even though no one can explain them. In due course, if the offending foods are eaten continually, reactions tend to be less severe but more prolonged and have a habit of running into the next reaction. The symptoms have become masked.

Other features at the time: Ann no longer enjoyed her kids, although she managed to keep going and do what was needed. Eventually they stopped showing her things they had done at school. She was not interested. She used to be; in the past she had always taken a great pride in everything they did.

To make matters worse, she had started developing headaches, and often went to bed with one. What with her loss of interest in sex, Ken really began to think their marriage was falling apart. To him, the headache was 'just the old excuse'. However, there was nothing he could do about it. He certainly was not the sort of man to force his attentions on his wife. He tried to get Ann to talk about it, and she assured him that she still loved him and that it was not his fault. She could not really talk about it – she did not know what to say.

As the body is trying to cope with food allergies, new symptoms often emerge, possibly caused by a new food allergy. Headache is an extremely common symptom of a reaction to one or more foods, as is loss of libido.

Anne goes to a doctor: Ken said she went to her G.P. a few times, but never really told him what was discussed. Ann told him that once the doctor had asked if she was feeling all right because she looked a little pale and low in spirits. She said she had made some sort of excuse about having just got over a heavy cold, but she did not think the doctor was convinced. He had asked her if she might be anaemic and did she have heavy periods? Even though she had said 'No', she let him take a blood sample to check. It came back perfectly normal. Actually, she did not go back to find out the result. She assumed he would get in touch if there was anything wrong. They only found out the result later.

Ann was lucky to have a caring doctor. Because of the large number of patients each G.P. has on his panel, it is extremely difficult to spend enough time with each patient. No G.P. can be expected to do anything if the patient does not ask for help and explain the problem. At this point, Ann's doctor was probably becoming suspicious that all was not well with her, hence the blood sample. It would take a few minutes to do and give him a chance to ask a few more questions. Besides, he was right, she may have been a little anaemic so the test was worthwhile doing anyway.

She should have been more open: She wished now she had been more open with her doctor. He was a kind, caring man and she knew how lucky she was to be on his list. So many of her friends complained about their doctors, although she had not taken much interest in their opinions. It is always so difficult to open up your heart to your doctor when you cannot really work out yourself what it is all about. It would be so much easier with a broken leg or discharging ear, or something obvious, but her symptoms were so vague. What with all those kids coughing in the waiting-room and that poor lady with such terrible arthritis in her hands, how could she take up so much of her doctor's time when there were so many ill patients for him to see?

Symptoms that don't really fit into a neat pigeon hole are often a typical food allergy reaction.

Things get worse: So Ann did not do anything about herself for ages. There were times when she seemed to go into herself and shut the world out all together. They did not take a holiday that year and Ken started coming home from work later and later. Presumably he was trying to avoid her. In a round about way this helped him get his promotion. Despite all this, Ann managed to keep the house going. Something inside her told her that was important. If she could not manage her house, she really was at the end. Maybe it was pride. She did not know; she did not really care.

One day: One day when Ken came home around 8.00 pm, he had to use his own key to let himself into the house. Despite everything else Ann had always let him in herself, but not tonight. The kids were getting ready for bed, but Ann was in the toilet being sick. Apparently she had been sick and had had diarrhoea for much of the day, and had crawled in and out of bed, seemingly running to the toilet every half an hour or so. She had even moved into the spare bedroom since it was nearer the bathroom. A friend had fetched the kids from school. Ken got cross with her for not ringing him. She broke down and wept.

The gastro-enteritis could have been the beginning of things really going wrong in her body. Up to now her symptoms were mainly food reactions. Her infection will have cleared her bowel of friendly organisms and made it easy for candida to gain a strong foothold.

Ken rings the doctor for advice: As usual, he was willing to come round, but Ken promised to ring if she got worse. The doctor came the next day. Ann had had a pretty disturbed night and so had Ken, of course. He had insisted she move back into the main bedroom with him. He had wanted to keep an eye on her. The doctor confirmed what they both suspected, that she had picked up a bug somewhere and had got gastro-enteritis. In fact, one of the kids had felt a little sick the day before, and the next day the other started with diarrhoea. The doctor confirmed that quite a lot of his patients had much the same.

The doctor gave suitable advice and reassured her she would be up and about in a few days, but the bug left its mark on her. She became extremely weak, had a splitting headache, and was even more depressed and just could not face anything to eat. Ken asked the doctor to visit her again on the third day, as she seemed to be getting worse even though her stomach had settled. The kindly doctor examined her thoroughly and reassured them that this occasionally did happen to some people. He felt sure she would be better soon. He gave an injection to help her rest, which certainly seemed to help and she slept soundly until the next morning.

I commonly ask patients if they have ever had a tummy bug or something that put them off their food for a few days, and how did they feel? Ann's story is remarkably common, but the explanation is nearly always missed. By not eating because of the gastro-enteritis, Ann started to develop withdrawal symptoms. Typically the symptoms of depression, headache, aches and pains etc get worse by the third day of a fast. At this stage a strong injection can work wonders, as it did with Ann. It covers the peak of the withdrawal symptoms.

Ann feels better: When the doctor came the next day, even he was surprised how effective his injection had been. Ann was sitting up in bed, smiling all over her face and claiming she had not felt so good for a long time. She was merely waiting for his say-so before getting up. The next day she felt even better.

Once the withdrawal peak is over, it is amazing how quickly symptoms disappear. It is just like the crisis of an infection from the old days before antibiotics became available. Within 24 hours or less symptoms can almost disappear, having been very severe. At this stage patients often comment how well they are and that they had forgotten what it was like to feel so well.

Ann starts to eat: They were advised that she should start eating again very cautiously. She had not had anything to eat for four days and felt she had lost pounds in weight, but her stomach would probably be a little delicate for a day or two longer. So she had some steamed fish and a little boiled rice, and felt fine.

The choice of foods Ann broke her 'fast' with were obviously not ones she had previously been reacting to.

Ann gets up: The next day she got up with the birds, and had the housework done before 8.30 am. It was a Sunday and Ken could not believe his eyes when he woke up to see her smiling down at him with a cup of tea in her hand. This was the Ann of old he had almost forgotten existed. How could she change so much after such a debilitating tummy bug? Maybe she had had time to think things through and decided to pull herself together. Anyway, he certainly was not going to rock the boat by talking about it just yet. It was obvious how she felt. She looked a different person altogether.

Maybe Ann felt so well that she did not even bother with a cup of tea herself. If she had, she may well have had a reaction that morning.

The visit: Ann reminded Ken that they were going to her parents after lunch. Ken had forgotten, what with Ann being so ill. She assured him she was perfectly well enough to go out and it was a beautiful day for a drive. Ann made them all a good salad for lunch and then they set off in the car. Ann had always done her best to be cheerful whenever she visited her parents, although it had been a great effort. But even they commented on how well she was looking. Her mum said she must have lost a stone in weight, and then her tummy bug illness was explained. They all agreed she must be fit and healthy to have got over it so quickly and so well.

Ann's lunch presumably consisted of an allergy-free salad. A lot of 'weight' carried by a person suffering from food allergies is fluid. If a normal woman were to go on a five day fast, she would lose approximately five pounds in weight. An 'overweight' food allergic patient may lose ten to fourteen pounds during the five day fast. It is simply the loss of previously-accumulated allergic fluid, plus natural loss from not eating. Ann would also have lost fluid in her vomit and diarrhoea. It is therefore not surprising that Ann's parents thought she must have lost so much weight.

Ann starts to feel unwell: Around 4.00 pm, as was their habit, Ann helped her mother make tea and sandwiches. She was in a bubbly mood. She talked excitedly about this and that, and her mother kept admiring her bounce and energy, especially after having been so ill. They took the trays out into the garden, set everything out properly and called the others to join them.

No one particularly noticed Ann become quieter as the meal progressed, nor thought anything of it when she slipped quietly into the house. But when she had not come back after 15 minutes, her mum went to look for her and found her upstairs in her old bedroom crying her eyes out. For five minutes she was unconsolable, and then Ken found them. Within minutes the whole family was round her.

It is most likely Ann started to react to the bread of the sandwiches. Remember, she had probably not eaten any bread or wheat based products since the start of her tummy bug. So by eating bread on the sixth day of avoidance, she was in a state of maximum sensitivity. Reactions to wheat can be a bit slow in some people, although they can be just as quick as with any other food at times. Ann probably started feeling unwell within 10 to 15 minutes of her first sandwich, and 15 minutes later her reaction was at its peak. In fact, the reaction may have been started by a cup of tea with mother while getting everyone else's ready.

Ken fears the worst: Gradually she calmed down a little, complained of a headache and said she felt tired. She also had a pain in the lower part of her tummy and it had hurt her to pass water. Her mum gave her some paracetemol and told her to get into bed. Obviously she had overdone it after being so ill during the week. Everyone agreed that that was the explanation. In half an hour Ann was asleep. Apart from someone saying they hoped she would soon be better, no one particularly mentioned Ann when they talked about other things. But poor Ken. He had seen it all before. He did not know what to do or say. He had been so pleased with Ann's transformation of the morning. She had been just like the girl he had married 13 years ago. Sadly, it had lasted a mere few hours. Would it ever come back again?

After Ann's typical reaction of crying and depression had begun to wane, she started to complain of other symptoms such as fatigue, headache and cystitis. After eating a food to which the patient is sensitive, not all symptoms appear at the same time. Despite the different timing, it is interesting that Ann eventually produced her three main symptoms, plus a first for cystitis. If she had been questioned closely, there could well have been others such as aches and pains all over the body. A careful observer would probably have noticed that Ann did not pass any water for quite a long time, and that she had become a bit swollen again. She may also have become thirsty. She would have been re-accumulating allergic fluid into her tissues.

Ann's mother helps: As it was so obvious to Ann's mother that Ann had not really had enough time to recover properly, she offered to come over the next day while Ann stayed in bed a few more days. True to her word, she arrived at 8.00 am the next morning to help Ken get the kids ready and off to school. Ann, meanwhile, stayed in bed. She had been up many times during the night with what she decided must be cystitis. She also still felt pretty awful.

It is quite possible the family had brought her up a cup of tea every so often, so keeping her cystitis going.

Ann has tests: Ann's mother asked the doctor to call some time during the day. He examined her thoroughly and sent a specimen of her urine to the laboratory. In the meantime he gave her a prescription for an antibiotic to help clear it up. When he came back in a couple of days he was pleased to see her feeling better, but said the laboratory test had not showed up anything special to explain her attack of cystitis. Anyway, now that she was better for the antibiotic, she should finish the five day course and get up when she felt well enough.

An antibiotic is often not necessary for cystitis, as in Ann's case where no infection was present. In fact it probably helped to kill off any of her normal bowel flora still surviving after the gastro-enteristis.

Ann remains unwell: When Ann seemed not to have fully recovered a week later, her mother went down with her to the doctor. She was given a tonic, but it did not really do much for her. She remained dispirited, fatigued, and achey all over, and complained of headaches. At times she would cry but not for long though; just long and often enough for everyone to start getting worried about her. A few months after the tummy bug Ken told Ann's parents that she had really been like this for at least two years, and on thinking it over he had seen a few signs for quite some time before that.

Having had such a severe reaction, and not taken any antidote (sodium and potassium bicarbonate or Epsom Salts), the reaction inevitably went on and on for a number of days. On occasions such a reaction can take weeks. Ann probably kept the reaction going by having a number of foods, such as bread and tea, not realizing them to be the cause of her symptoms.

Ann sees her doctor again: When Ann next went to see her doctor, his attitude had changed. He started talking about her family life, her home and her relationships with Ken. She did her best to be honest with him, but it was not difficult for him to see how flat her mood was, and how unexcited she was about anything in the future. She certainly did not have any plans nor were they even considering their next holiday, or anything like that. The doctor asked her to come back in one week, with Ken.

At the next visit to the surgery, Ann was given a prescription for something to 'lift her mood'. It had a strange sounding name, but it was not like Valium or Librium, they were told. Ken was not convinced. He asked a pharmacist friend of his to find out what they were.

They turned out to be a new drug just on the market. They were basically an anti-depressant but could help any anxiety that was accompanying the depression. Depressed Ann might well be, but Ken did not think that she was suffering from anxiety.

You can see the change in her doctor's approach. He is now thinking of psychological factors, and tries a tranquillizer of sorts.

Life on tranquillizers: Ann knew her doctor was trying to help her, but she did not like the effect the new capsules had on her. The only word she could think of was that they made her feel like a 'zombie' and even more tired than before. Ann had never really had any difficulty with sleep, in fact she tended to sleep too much yet always felt tired. These capsules made it impossible for her to get up to get the kids ready for school, so Ken had to do it.

She found it extremely difficult to concentrate, and within a week the kids had told Ken that mum had had two near misses in the car fetching them from school, something that had never happened before. This frightened Ken who told her to stop the capsules at once. Her doctor felt he ought to try some others to find one that suited her. In the meantime her mum would temporarily move in with them to fetch and carry the children.

But it was no good. Nothing seemed to help her, and all the drugs that the doctor tried made her feel worse, some more so than others. In the end he arranged for Ann to see a psychistrist at the local hospital. She was lucky that she only had to wait six weeks.

The failure of psychotropic drugs (used for psychological symptoms) to help a patient, and more particularly if they make her worse, is a strong indication that she **does** *have a food allergy.*

The tablets change: After a long chat with the specialist, Ann was given a prescription for some different tablets, and told not to eat certain foods like cheese and marmite. He gave her a list. Ken later found out these were mono-amine oxidase inhibitors (MAOI), drugs specifically used for depression.

The only time most psychiatrists suggest an alteration in a patient's diet is when they use these powerful drugs.

The decline: They seemed okay for the first few days,but within a week she felt 'drugged' and could not concentrate or think straight. Simple jobs like cooking scrambled eggs on toast became a mammoth task. She could not remember what to do with the eggs when they were cooked, and forgot to turn the oven off. It seemed that she would never tolerate any of these drugs.

In-patient: When Ann visited the psychiatrist a month later, he invited her to come into hospital for observation. She did not really like the idea but agreed. A week later someone from the hospital rang her and said there was a bed for her that Sunday afternoon.

Nothing much happened for the first two days. She found the ward old and smelly. There were some rather odd people in the hospital, and Ann felt sure she was not as bad as they were. Because she could not tolerate any drug, they gave her shock treatment under a general anaesthetic. The idea scared her, but she talked to a friendly lady in the bed opposite who had just had it done and she seemed okay. What Ann did not realize was that she had lost her memory for things that had happened recently. The same happened to Ann. When she came round from the anaesthetic, she could not remember why she was in hospital, and she hardly recognized Ken when he visited her that evening.

Ann had a course of six treatments, and seemed to brighten up more after each one. She spent about two weeks in hospital, and was discharged home in a far better frame of mind than when she went into hospital. Even though she was not as bright and happy as she was when she got married, for example, the treatment certainly seemed to have helped her. At least she did not have to take those awful pills. The psychiatric social worker visited her at home, and she saw the specialist again a couple of times, then he discharged her.

It was probably nine months later that things started to go gradually wrong again. It was difficult to put a finger on it, but in retrospect she remembered starting a few headaches and getting a bit more tired. In particular, however, life once again became more mundane and boring and she lost interest in things. Even after leaving hospital she had remained a little forgetful – the silliest things like where she had put her car keys or her purse. Her sex drive had never really returned. Ken had tried to make love to her, but he had not managed to rouse her much at all. In fact she developed cystitis on two occasions after intercourse.

Sometimes a particular treatment may actually help the body to tolerate food allergies better. For example, some drugs have anti-allergic properties which can themselves be helpful. All too often, however, the relief is temporary, as the cause of the symptoms, food allergies, has not been removed. Symptoms tend to creep in again unless something dramatic like a shock or bereavement, etc. happens – when the deterioration tends to be more rapid.

Continuing depression: Arrangements were made for Ann to see the psychiatrist again. Reluctantly, he suggested that another course of shock treatment would be worth trying, as Ann refused to try drugs again. But when Ken asked if they could expect any lasting benefit from another course the specialist was not able to say yes or no. In some cases it could be very effective, in others not so good. The only thing to do was to try it and see.

Ken, however, wanted to know more. As he pointed out, Ann had no reason to be depressed. It was explained to him that Ann suffered from endogenous depression, i.e. the depression was coming from within herself. Psychoanalysis could probably help her come to terms with her problem, or maybe under hypnosis she would be able to declare what she was concerned about. Something in the past, like a relationship, the harbouring of a sexual desire for her father, or possibly a glimpse of her mother and father in bed together many years ago, may have left a deep imprint on her subconscious mind. Perhaps it was something like this that made her produce symptoms of cystitis after intercourse, to make Ken feel guilty so that he would not try to make love to her. Only now in adulthood had something triggered it all off, causing her depression.

This is a typical Freudian explanation, of the sort that has been used for years by psychiatrists to explain symptoms such as Ann's. Perhaps it applies to some patients, but its concepts are so unrealistic to many ordinary doctors, and certainly to non-doctors. It is interesting that Freud himself maintained that a biochemical approach to mental symptoms would become more important in the future. He thought that in the 19th century! Modern psychiatry does not seem to have caught up.

Shock treatment: So Ann had her second course of shock treatment, but this time it did not help so much. It made her memory even worse. When an extended course was suggested they decided not to have it, and took her home. That was a year ago.

About six months ago, Ann was given a course of antibiotics for a bout of tonsilitis. While it helped her throat, she got an attack of thrush. A couple of days later she had cystitis. Once again the urine test was negative, but her doctor said it was because the germ had presumably been killed by the antibiotic. It was just that the symptoms were a bit late coming out. He did wonder, however, if the thrush had anything to do with it, so gave her some pessaries to insert every night for a week.

Doctors seldom seem able to track down the cause of tonsillitis, and far too readily resort to antibiotics. Simple measures like gargling in warm salt water and taking large doses of vitamin C should be tried first. **Food allergies** *are not considered. This time the antibiotic definitely precipitated the attack of thrush.*

Upset stomach: For some time after that, Ann's tummy seemed to trouble her every so often. It wasn't much at first, but gradually she would have wind, slight pain and occasional diarrhoea, not always all together. She felt food upset her, but not every time she had a meal.

A colony of Candida albicans had now become established in her bowel and was making its presence felt.

Cystitis and sex: On more than one occasion Ann had developed a nasty attack of cystitis after they had made love. Strangely enough it had occurred when she really hadn't wanted to have sex, but she had done it to oblige Ken. On other occasions when she had been more willing, she had seemed all right. Ken had felt rather guilty and had wondered if the psychiatrist was right after all. However, he decided it was pure coincidence as she had had other attacks of cystitis without their making love.

What had really alarmed her was the first time she passed blood in her water. She thought her period had started, then remembered she wasn't due for another two weeks. In a panic she called the doctor who gave her an antibiotic and arranged for her to see the specialist. Unfortunately she also had thrush again.

The specialist organized a number of tests, including a cystoscopy, which all turned out OK. They felt reassured but were still somewhat mystified. The specialist suggested a long term course of a urinary antiseptic, but, after three weeks when Ann had another attack, she gave them up. Since then she had had a number of attacks, some not too bad, others agonizing.

They read books: It was around this time that Ken was talking to a friend about Ann, how no one seemed able to explain to him in a way that satisfied him why this had all happened to her. To Ken it just did not make sense. Ann really had no cause for depression and he did not accept the psychiatrist's theory about something in her past now coming out. Could her mind be playing tricks on her? Was she really able to produce an attack of cystitis to keep him away from her?

Ken's friend said his wife had had a similar experience, though not so bad as Ann's, and they had found out that it was instant coffee that had made her so tired and gave her a headache. They had read about it first in a health magazine. To Ken it seemed a bit of an odd idea, that coffee could make you tired. Surely coffee gave most people a lift *when* they were tired.

Ken's reaction was quite normal. It is true that coffee is a brain stimulant in certain circumstances. Once the patient has become addicted to coffee, without it she can become very tired. Another coffee picks her up, but she then goes very low again until the next cup. The only way to break this vicious circle is to give up coffee altogether, suffer the withdrawal symptoms (which is not so difficult once you know what is causing it all), and return to normal.

Food allergies: By coincidence, however, Ann's mum read an article in a daily paper about 'food allergies', which explained how some people could develop migraine, headaches, fatigue, depression, cystitis, aches and pains, constipation, diarrhoea, and all sorts of conditions just by eating certain foods, often the ones they most commonly ate. The article mentioned a number of books to read on the subject, so they bought a couple, and realized that Ann's problems could well be explained on the same basis.

When I first saw Ann there were even fewer clinical ecologists than there are now. Many people still rely on information in books such as this one, and magazine articles to help themselves get better. Doctors seem the slowest of all to hear about these ideas, let alone accept them and put them into practice. Don't orthodox doctors ever read books and magazine articles on **health**, *as opposed to* **disease**? *Probably not.*

They find a Clinical Ecologist: Their main problem was to be sure, and, though some of the suggestions made in the books seemed to be worth trying, they felt a bit out of their depth and preferred to find someone who could guide them. It is all very well altering your diet, they thought, but what if things go wrong? So they wrote to an organization mentioned in one of the books, which gave them a list of doctors practising Clinical Ecology. That is how they found their way to me.

They come to see me: To obtain such a detailed history from a patient can take a long time, and it does not all come out of the first interview. At the second visit, bits and pieces are often added to throw additional light on the problem. Ann thought that what she had described should be quite sufficient for any doctor, so she was surprised when I asked what other symptoms she suffered from.

Many doctors themselves become concerned when presented with a patient suffering from multiple symptoms. They therefore rapidly come to the conclusion that it is 'all in the mind'. Patients in their turn soon learn not to reveal too many symptoms all at once, tending to describe their most serious problems or the ones they feel the doctor is interested in. In addition, because some symptoms are so important, they may consider other symptoms not to be important or relevant.

Other symptoms: After a little prompting, she talked about a number of other symptoms. There had been times when she felt as though she was coming down with 'flu, because she ached all over, bones, muscles and joints, but without any signs of a fever. The aches might only last a few hours, but occasionally up to a few days. She would just be aware that they had gone. She supposed she must have got used to them.

Typical allergic symptoms of involvement of muscles and joints. If they become the major symptoms they can lead to a diagnosis of arthritis so rheumatoid and osteoarthritis may well respond to this approach.

Ann puts on weight: Perhaps because she was so lacking in energy and all the joys of life, she had not been too concerned about her personal appearance. Sure, she had kept herself clean, but she had not been too bothered about her gradual increase in weight. Before she had gone into hospital the first time, her weight had been as high as $12^1/_2$ st, and she must have looked awful, especially as she was only five foot four inches tall.

Much of Ann's weight gain would have been the accumulation of allergic fluid.

Symptoms admitted but not volunteered: Patients often feel embarrassed at their many complaints, but, as I usually explain, it is the rule rather than the exception to have multiple symptoms. Because they are not the main symptoms worrying a patient, others may well exist and complete the picture, so it is always worthwhile having a check list to go through. Using such a check list, it appeared that Ann had occasionally felt dizzy and often had catarrh, though not always when she thought the 'flu was coming on. She suffered occasional pins and needles, usually in her hands, which occurred most commonly at night, when she might also develop cramp in her legs. Despite being overweight she seemed to have poor circulation for her hands were always cold.

On one or two nights per week she would have palpitations for about five to 10 minutes shortly after getting into bed. At times she could hear her heart pounding in her head, and once or twice she thought her head was going to burst. Apart from the tummy troubles she had already described, there were times when she felt so bloated that the discomfort almost amounted to pain, and it made her breathing difficult. If was unquestionably worse during the week before her period, but it could be just as bad at other times of the month. Most of her symptoms tended to be worse premenstrually.

Premenstrual hormonal imbalances can make a woman more food sensitive. On the other hand food allergies can cause premenstrual tension.

Constipation: When asked if she ever had diarrhoea, she managed a weak smile and said 'A chance would be a fine thing'. All her life she had struggled with her bowels, and had regularly to resort to Epsom Salts or something similar. She had read that bran was good for the bowels and had tried it. If anything it had made her constipation worse.

The accumulation of allergic fluid in her bowel wall as an allergic reaction to wheat may have caused the constipation. In the initial stages the reaction may be more of a direct irritant on the lining of the intestine, only to become an allergic one in due course. Milk and wheat are common causes of constipation in children and adults alike.

Vaginal discharge: Vaginal discharge had come and gone, some days being quite heavy, that is apart from the thrush. Much of the time, however, the discharge was watery but seemed more than she ought to have. Only on rare occasions did it make her sore or itchy; but it soon went.

While Ann's vaginal discharge may have been caused by candida without always causing typical features of thrush, changes in quality and quantity of vaginal discharge can occur with changing allergic states. Individual foods can be clearly found to cause or exacerbate vaginal discharge.

A weak bladder: As she had already explained, she had had quite a number of episodes of cystitis, although the doctor had seldom been able to demonstrate infection in her urine. She felt she must be developing a weak bladder or have a prolapse or something, because there were many nights when she had to get out of bed more than twice to go to the toilet to pass water. Some days she seemed to be going to the toilet almost every hour, and it became a family joke. If they went on a long car journey they would plan their stops around Ann's weak bladder. Then, for no obvious reason, it would all disappear and she seemed hardly to pass any water for days. In fact it was Ken who noticed this. He thought there was a connection between Ann stopping passing so much water and the development of a fit of depression. To be honest, she said, it was the cystitis that was now worrying her the most as it hurt so badly.

Many food-allergic patients have a smaller bladder than normal, presumably because the chronic irritation of an allergic type causes the muscles in the bladder wall to go into spasm. Hence such a patient cannot last so long and has to keep going to the toilet. At other times, if a patient is shedding allergic fluid, the bladder irritation may go, but now there will be a lot more fluid to excrete. To the patient these two situations may be the same. With the former, however, there will be the frequent passage of smaller amounts of urine, often with a little discomfort and a feeling of never quite having emptied the bladder. With the latter there may be slightly less frequent visits but the passage of normal or increased amount of urine.

Ann's mother helps with details: Right from birth Ann apparently cried a lot. She seemed to have colic all the time, and was a very sicky baby. At first it was put down to the jaundice, but when her colour cleared and the crying went on it was diagnosed as 'three month colic'. As the name implies, Ann's mother was told it would stop at three months.

Colic and being a 'sicky baby' are highly suggestive of a cow's milk allergy. A bottle-fed baby is usually weaned far earlier than a breast-fed one. In Ann's case this meant cutting down on the total amount of cow's milk she was being given. It also may have coincided with the development of stage two, of the stage of tolerance.

A reaction to milk: With Ann at home, a very helpful health visitor recommended a different milk. The first one they tried seemed to make her worse, but the second satisfied her more, or certainly did not seem to upset her so much. She could not remember what its name was.

By changing milks round one can often be found to which the baby is less allergic. The difference in the process of manufacture may alter the chemical nature of one milk more than another. Some adults find they can have tinned milk but not ordinary milk.

Projectile vomiting: Around three months old, solids like rusks were started which at first seemed to help the colic. But then Ann started to vomit more. At times it was projectile. The distance she could actually propel the vomit was quite extraordinary. Even more strange was the fact that it did not seem to upset her. Her doctor referred her to a specialist because he thought she might have congenital pyloric stenosis – a condition in which the muscles at the junction between the stomach and the next part (called the duodenum) are abnormally developed. That diagnosis was not confirmed. In time, and with suitable treatment, the projectile vomiting seemed to settle, but Ann remained a sicky baby.

The projectile vomiting probably started with the introduction of wheat-based products. Wheat and milk allergies seem so commonly to occur together.

A baby's bowel habits: Although Ann had laughed when I originally asked her if she had ever had diarrhoea, her mother said that, as a baby, her stools were very loose, foul smelling and a bit difficult to flush away during the first three months when she had had the colic. Thereafter, once the vomiting had started, she had become constipated. And had seemed to stay that way for the rest of her life.

Milk allergy in a baby often leads to loose stools, amongst other things. The constipation that often develops after weaning may be either a change from an irritative effect of milk initially to an allergic one (hence producing different symptoms), or the direct allergic affect of the wheat, or both.

A snuffly baby: From very early on Ann had also been a snuffly baby. It had never been much, and no one really bothered about it. So many other babies seemed the same way. During the years before starting school Ann had quite a lot of colds and ear trouble, but it was when she actually started school that she seemed to pick up everything. She must have been absent from school many weeks during her first two years as a junior, and was taken regularly to the doctor for antibiotics. In the end she had her tonsils and adenoids removed when she was seven and a half, which was a great help. Nevertheless she was still prone to throat and ear infections for the next few years, even though the operation had made a lot of difference.

A history of snuffles, tonsillitis, regular sore throats or colds or frequent ear trouble are regular features of food allergic patients, commonly to cow's milk. Whilst these problems may not be too bad before the child goes to school, the additional burden of all the coughs and colds and infections brought in by other children is too much for the reacting child, who seems to catch everything in sight. The non-allergic can usually cope perfectly well. Sometimes removal of tonsils and adenoids removes the seat of a lot of infecton, which has been keeping things going all the time. For some patients the operation makes very little difference.

During her teens: Ann went through a good phase around 11, although she put on a bit of weight. In those days, school milk was free and everyone thought how funny it was that Ann drank so much. Some of her friends did not like milk, so Ann always drank their share, which was presumably why she was a little overweight. In the village where they lived, her mother's milk bill was the biggest, and Ann had most of it.

During her teens Ann was probably into stage two of adaptation. She was quite clearly drinking too much milk, and was probably moving into the third stage, the stage of addiction. The different stages can sometimes last for years. Her extra weight may have been her bad diet, the accumulation of allergic fluid without symptoms, or both.

Late periods: During her early teens, Ann seemed quite happy with life and had no particular problems when her periods started a little late at 14. Like most of her friends, she probably ate too many crisps and sweets and drank too much pop, and did not much care for vegetables. Somewhere in her middle teens she started developing a few headaches, but they were put down to the stress of studying for her exams. Her eye test was normal.

There is some evidence that late onset of periods may occur in a teenager who is zinc deficient. To make things worse she was probably eating too much junk food which has been virtually stripped of all its essential vitamins and minerals. An 'average' diet may only contain 8 mg to 13 mg of zinc per day, but our daily requirement is 15 mg, and more during stress. 20 mg are needed during preganancy and 25 mg during breast feeding. Zinc is essential to over one hundred enzyme functions, so any deficiency will mean that these enzymes will not be as efficient as they should be. The human body will therefore be working under par, setting a person up for allergic reactions later on. Her exams could have been an additional stress.

Having left school: Later in her teens she became fashion conscious and started to eat better. She lost over two stone and bought all the latest style clothes. She went to secretarial college for a year and landed a good job as personal assistant to the managing director of a local building firm. Through the job she met Ken and they got married when she was 20. Quite obviously she could remember her wedding day very well, but what upset her now was looking at their album of photographs. She was so slim – she remembered weighing herself on the morning of her wedding day – she was exactly eight stone. She could also remember how happy and energetic she was. She and Ken had gone on honeymoon ski-ing in Austria. Although she was not any good, she had skied every day and danced every evening. What a contrast her boundless energy was in those days to the way she felt now!

By taking her diet in hand, her nutritional status would have improved and she would have stopped eating certain foods to which she had previously reacted, but she probably did it all gradually. With a special goal in mind, such as a slim body, she would have put up with withdrawal symptoms, or may simply have forgotten all about them.

The contraceptive pill: Ann had gone onto the contraceptive pill a month before she and Ken had got married. Unlike some of her friends she had felt perfectly well on it. The only thing that happened was that she found she needed a slightly larger bra. As with most women her periods became absolutely regular, were two days shorter than before, and she had no period pains whatsoever. She felt lucky. She knew some of her friends had had to stop because the pill had made them so ill. In fact she put on about a stone in the first year; it just crept on gradually.

Her improved diet may have only just corrected her nutritional status to normal. Unfortunately the contraceptive pill has a bad affect upon a number of essential substances, causing a fall of zinc, vitamin C and vitamin B6 in particular. So Ann's improved health was easily upset again by taking the pill, even if she still kept to what she thought was a good diet.

Changing pills: She and Ken had decided not to start a family for a few years, so she stayed on the pill. About three years after they had been married, Ann realized she was losing interest in her job. She also found that life was not nearly so exciting as it had been when they were first married. She did not seem to have as much energy, and she became uninterested in sex. About six months later she was due for her annual contraceptive pill renewal, and her doctor asked her quite a number of questions. When she revealed a few problems he swopped her pill for another one. After two months he tried again, and this time she felt a little better. Actually, she exaggerated how well she felt because she did not want to keep bothering him for something so trivial.

Loss of interest in sex is a sign not only of zinc and or vitamin B6 deficiency, but is commonly found in allergic patients. Being such a private subject, however, it is often not mentioned. Changing the pill round can sometimes make a difference, but usually not in the long run.

Starting a family: At the age of 25, they decided to start a family, so Ann stopped the pill. Despite not feeling very energetic or having much interest in sex, Ann knew it was about time she got pregnant. Having made up her mind, she found her interest in sex increasing and her energy levels rising. She felt she had made the right decision. Within two months of stopping the pill she knew she was pregnant. She and Ken were delighted.

Ann felt better probably **because** *she stopped the contraceptive pill.*

A miscarriage: Three months later Ann had a miscarriage. It was a terrible blow and upset her very much. Her doctor told her that the best thing to do was to get pregnant again as soon as possible. So she took his advice and it was not long before she was pregnant again. The first clue she had was morning sickness. Despite the nausea she was delighted. Unfortunately her sickness got worse and by the end of the first month she was vomiting two or three times every morning. She lost her appetite and started to feel miserable again.

There is now a considerable weight of evidence that women should be off the contraceptive pill for a minimum of six months **before** *conceiving. Foresight, the Association for the Promotion of Pre-Conceptual Care, gives advice to couples on 'preparing for pregnancy'. Miscarriages at around three months, the most common time, can probably be prevented by taking sensible steps before conception.*

The advice to get pregnant straightaway was definitely wrong. The reason Ann had a miscarriage should have been corrected, i.e. she should have stayed off the pill and should have been given zinc and vitamin B6 supplements. Her diet should also have been checked for its adequacy. However, Ann got away with it, she kept her next pregnancy, but at great cost to herself, for the baby took all the nutrients it required. The vomiting meant her food intake was severely reduced so she had no chance to replenish her depleted nutrient stores.

A visit to the clinic: The vomiting got worse, and at times she could not even keep down water. Ann thought that three months was the normal time to attend the ante-natal clinic for the first time, but Ken took her along to the doctor when she was only six weeks. He scolded her for not letting him know earlier and gave her something to settle her down. He assured her it would not harm the baby.

Although it would have been better to try zinc and vitamin B6 or magnesium to stop the sickness, it was quite reasonable for her doctor to stop it with a drug, thought to be safe. Her mineral deficiencies would have otherwise become even worse, even though her doctor did not realize she would have benefitted from supplements. A doctor needs to balance the possible risk to the fetus from the drug against the dangers continuous vomiting might inflict upon mother and baby.

The pregnancy: Ann was not happy at the idea of taking tablets, so she avoided them for a week, but was so bad she took one. It seemed to work so she stuck to it for a week. Every time she stopped the pills the sickness came back with a vengeance. Finally, at five months, the sickness settled and she remained quite well until she was due. In fact she went two weeks over and had to be induced. The labour lasted fourteen hours and was quite difficult, but by all accounts nowhere near as bad as when her mum had her.

Post-natal depression: To cap it all she felt depressed for two months after the birth of her baby son whom she had to bottle-feed. She was not sure why, and an appointment was made for her to see a psychiatrist. Ken thought it was to nip it in the bud, or possibly to frighten her into pulling herself together. In the end the appointment was cancelled as she settled sufficiently well. But she remained uninterested in sex for at least a year afterwards.

The difficult labour and post-natal depression are further evidence of a zinc deficiency. Once the demands of the baby inside her were no longer a drain on her own body stores, and she began to eat, her zinc levels may have improved somewhat. Had she breast-fed, her post-natal depression might have gone on longer. However, women who are depressed seldom breast-feed for long, as they can't be bothered. Rejection of the baby is another part of post-natal depression.

Another pregnancy: Almost exactly 15 months after the boy was born, Ann got pregnant again, and, apart from a few minor problems, the pregnancy proceeded reasonably well and she gave birth to a girl, also two weeks late having had to be induced again. This time the labour was not so difficult. Apart from being a little low for a week afterwards, she did not have any depression.

Her comparative zinc deficiency may have persisted, but it is amazing how the body can sometimes adapt to a less-than-perfect nutritional state. In any case she did not go back onto the contraceptive pill.

After the children were born: Despite never being as energetic as she had been when they were first married, Ann settled into her task as a housewife and mother. She had given up her job when she had become pregnant properly for the first time, and never thought of getting a job again. As with so many of her friends, she found some days boring and hankered after a little more spare time, but she accepted her responsibilities. She was certainly feeling better than she had felt when she was 23 or 24.

Presumably because she was more tired looking after the house and the children, and because she was no longer stimulated by the job she used to have, she found she had little interest in sex, although they did make love occasionally. Ann never went onto the pill again. She thought it may not have been too good for her in the past. She had read a few magazine articles that suggested a possible link between the pill and depression. In any case, she did not see much point in taking the pill regularly for the odd episode of love-making.

And so it was that she gradually lost interest in things around her, developed a few headaches, seemed depressed for no reason, suffered from cystitis every so often, and she came to the point where I first saw her.

In the end, all her dietary indiscretions, food allergies and incomplete nutritional status gradually caught up with her.

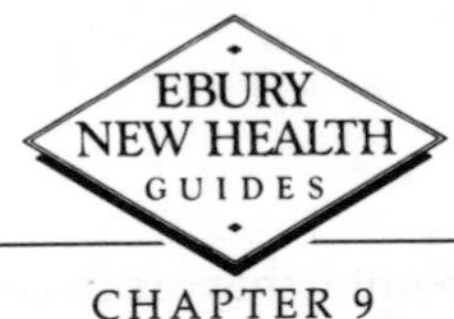

CHAPTER 9

TREATING CYSTITIS

UNDOUBTEDLY the best way for the sufferer from recurrent cystitis to be helped is to seek the advice of a physician specializing in clinical ecology and nutritional medicine. Sadly, however, such medically-qualified practitioners are all too thin on the ground, and the majority of those with such an interest are in private practice. General practitioners are becoming more interested in this approach to ill health, but they only see patients on their own panel.

The few hospital doctors who are enthusiastic about clinical ecology have to continue to operate within the normal mechanisms of the health service. Although they may want to analyze every patient they see in this way, the number of patients they have to see in each outpatient session makes it very difficult to do full justice to these ideas. I will therefore assume that a woman suffering from chronic cystitis will have to 'go it alone' and do for herself whatever she can.

It should be clear by now that I am suggesting that something in your diet is not only making you generally unwell, but is also causing your cystitis. The problem is to find out which food or foods. There are two areas to consider first. Is there a particular 'food' like tea, orange, milk or wheat, for example, that is having a specific affect upon your bladder, either irritating it via the urine or the blood stream, or is your present diet keeping the mould/yeast organism candida going? Or both?

The problem can be tackled in different ways. Think about your lifestyle. Do you have children to look after? Are you out at work? How difficult would it be to take food everywhere you go if you go onto a strict diet? When should you start? Is there a method you like the sound of and which you think you could cope with? Do you need help from family or friends? Do you need advice from a dietician?

This section on treatment describes various ways in which you can change what you are eating and drinking in an attempt to find out what is causing your cystitis. Often the simplest approach is the best and easiest. Each method has its advantages and disadvantages, and I cannot possibly dictate which one is best for you. That is why I have described five separate methods, although they are linked and could be combined in some way.

THE FOUR-DAY INVENTORY

One of the simplest things to do to begin with is to write down everything you eat, drink, or put into your mouth, for four consecutive days. Carry paper and pencil round with you and write down things AS YOU EAT THEM. Don't do it later – you are bound to forget. Do the inventory over a weekend, i.e. Friday, Saturday, Sunday, Monday, as you will therefore cover two week days (presumably work days) and two weekend days, although I appreciate that may not apply to everyone.

It does not matter what form the inventory takes. It could be like a chef preparing a menu of what is to be eaten over the next few days, which should be in amazing detail. Table 9.1 gives such a chart and is taken from one patient in particular, but with details from others that are worth including, to show how complete it should be. The four days of the inventory should be reasonably typical of your regular habits.

When I ask a person to do a four-day inventory, I remind them to include added salt, chewing gum, spoonfuls of sugar, sweets, chocolates, cigarettes, and all tablets, especially ones bought over the counter. When I talk about a dietary inventory most people only think of foods and drinks, yet they may have been chewing three or four packets of gum every day for years. In fact I found the blue colouring agent in someone's chewing gum to be the main cause of her symptoms (not cystitis). When she walked into my surgery with a piece in her mouth, I only half-jokingly asked her if she had put it on the chart she had been doing for me. That day I learned an object lesson.

Some people suffer from indigestion which they have had for so long they don't think it is important. In any case they take antacids from the chemist to keep it under control, so in fact don't suffer much in the way of symptoms. They keep their indigestion suppressed. To me, however, it is all part of the evidence that something is wrong and needs to be taken into consideration. Apart from that, if I advise a cow's milk-free diet, their tablets could contain lactose, so they may not improve. Writing out the inventory fully is extremely valuable and helps me pick up things I haven't thought of.

The other method of completing the four-day inventory is shown in table 9.2. Here, each item taken into the mouth is listed on the left, and the number of times it is taken in the day is indicated with a tick or a 1.

9·1 4-DAY DIETARY INVENTORY

	Friday 6th Dec.	Saturday 7th Dec.	Sunday 8th Dec.	Monday 9th Dec.
Early	0700 hrs. Mug of tea with milk.	0730–0930 hrs. 2 mugs of tea with milk.	0800–0930 hrs. 2 mugs of tea with milk.	0645 hrs. Mug of tea with milk.
Break-fast	0700 hrs. Cereal – Cornflakes, Harvest Crunch with milk and a sprinkle of demerara sugar. Fried egg on fried brown bread (cooked in vegetable oil). One mug instant coffee with cream and two teaspoonsful of white sugar. Toast, light textured brown, scrape of butter and marmalade.	1000 hrs. 2 rashers of grilled bacon, 2 grilled tomatoes, 2 slices of potato sautéed in vegetable oil. 2½ slices of toasted white bread, scrape of butter on each, honey. 2 mugs of ground coffee with cream and 2 teaspoonsful demerara sugar. 1230 hrs. 1 pint bitter, packet of plain crisps and a Mars Bar.	1000 hrs. Cereal – Cornflakes, Grape Nuts, top of the milk, sprinkle of demerara sugar. 1 large boiled egg. 2 large slices of wholemeal toast, scrape of butter, honey. 2 mugs of freshly ground coffee, cream and 2 demerara sugars.	0745 hrs. Cereal – Cornflakes with Harvest Crunch, sprinkle of demerara sugar and top of the milk. 1 rasher of bacon, grilled tomato. 1½ large slices of wholemeal toast, scrape of butter, marmalade. 1100 hrs. Mug of instant coffee, cream and 2 white sugars. 2 chocolate digestive biscuits.
Lunch	1315 hrs. Grilled smoked mackerel, squeeze of lemon, cauliflower, ½ pint cider, 1 Kit-Kat. 2 slices of chewing-gum.	1500 hrs. Grilled ham and cheese on toast (white bread). 1 banana. Thin slice of melon.	1245 hrs. 1 mug instant coffee, cream and 2 white sugars. 1330 hrs. 6 oz lentil and vegetable soup (home-made). 2 small slices white toast with cheese. 2 small mince pies with single cream.	1300 hrs. Fried whitebait (corn oil), squeeze of lemon, tinned carrots. ½ pint cider, packet of salt-and-vinegar crisps. 1 Kit-Kat.
p.m.	1515 hrs. Mug of instant coffee, 'Coffee Plus', 2 teaspoonsful of white sugar.		1600 hrs. Mug of instant coffee with cream and 2 teaspoonsful of demerara sugar. 4 oz bar Cadbury's Milk Chocolate.	1530 hrs. Cup of instant coffee with cream and 2 white sugars.
Tea	1730 hrs. 2 mugs of tea with milk and 2 teaspoonsful of white sugar. Slice of currant cake.	1730 hrs. 2 mugs of tea with milk. Small currant sponge. 1 cup cake. Small piece of chocolate sponge.	1820 hrs. Mug of tea with milk. Small currant sponge cup cake.	1730 hrs. Mug of tea with milk. Small piece of chocolate cake.
Supper	2000 hrs. ½ avocado containing chopped lettuce, oil and vinegar dressing. 7 oz turbot baked with garlic, olive oil, fresh lemon juice, 2 boiled potatoes, 1 grilled tomato and boiled broccoli. Coffee mousse with dollop of whipped fresh cream. ½ pint cider. 2 cups instant coffee, cream and 2 teaspoonsful demerara sugar.	2030 hrs. ½ pint lentil and vegetable soup (home-made), small slice of wholemeal bread. Smoked trout cold, tinned petit pois, salad (lettuce, cucumber, tomatoes and carrots). Mince pie (small) with single cream. Coffee mousse. ½ pint cider. Cup of instant coffee, whipped cream and 2 teaspoonsful white sugar.	1945 hrs. Cheese soufflé, 2 roast potatoes, 1 roast parsnip (both roasted in corn oil). Tinned petit pois. Salad (lettuce, tomatoes, green and red peppers, onion and carrots). Coffee mousse with single cream. 1 clementine. 4 oz Muscatel wine. 6 oz mineral water.	2000 hrs. Fish pie, potato slices baked in oil with herbs. Parsley sauce (packet). 2 mince pies with cream. 4 walnuts. 1 water biscuit, blue Cheshire cheese, scrape of butter, 2 sticks of celery. ½ pint mineral water.
Later	2200 hrs. 1 cup of instant coffee, milk and 2 sugars.	2215 hrs. Mug of ground coffee, cream and 2 white sugars.	2215 hrs. 1 cup of instant coffee with cream and 2 teaspoonsful of demerara sugar.	2200 hrs. Mug of instant coffee, cream and 2 teaspoonsful of white sugar.

Notes: mug = nearly ½ pint; cereal weighs about 2½ oz dry.

9·2 FOOD INTAKE OVER ONE WEEK

Day	Wed	Thurs	Fri	Sat	Sun	Mon	Tues
Date	6th Nov	7th Nov	8th Nov	9th Nov	10th Nov	11th Nov	12th Nov
Cup of tea	• • • • •	• • • • • •	• • • • • •	• • • • • • •	• • • • •	• • • • • •	• • • • • •
Cup of coffee	• • • •	• • •	• •	• • • • • •	• • • • • •	• • •	• • •
Teaspoonful of sugar per cup	• • • • • • • • •	• • • • • • • • •	• • • • • • • •	• • • • • • • • • • • • •	• • • • • • • • • • •	• • • • • • • • •	• • • • • • • •
Portions of milk	• • • •	• • •	• •	• • • • • •	• • • • • •	• • •	• • •
Glass of hot milk	•		•	• •	• •	•	•
Chocolate-covered biscuits	• •	• •	• •	• • •	• •	• •	• •
Slice of bread (white)	• • • •	• •	• •	• • •	• • • •	• •	• • •
Butter	• • • •	• •	• •	• • •	• • • •	• •	• • •
Cake	•		•		•	•	
Beef	•				•		
Eggs	•		•				•
Whole orange	•		•	•	•		•
Orange juice				• •	• •		
Orange squash	•	•	•				
Cabbage	•		•		•		
Carrots		•	•			•	•
Broccoli				•			
Rice	•			•			•
Potatoes		•	•		•	•	
Added salt	• • •	• • •	• • •	• •	• • • •	• •	• •
Bar of chocolate	•	•	•	• •	• •	•	•
Extend this column onto another sheet to include as many foods and drinks you take during the seven days.							

Make a chart like this for yourself. Put the names of each item in the left-hand column, and the day and date at the top of the columns. Put a • or a tick in the column for each day when you have a particular item. In the above example, the patient had five cups of tea and four cups of coffee on Wednesday 6th November, but seven cups of tea and six cups of coffee on the Saturday. Note that she had one teaspoonful of sugar in each cup, and therefore had sixty-eight teaspoonful of sugar in the week, let alone the hidden sugar in other parts of her diet. She had one bar of chocolate every day, but two on the Saturday and Sunday, as well as at least two chocolate-covered biscuits each day. She added salt at most meals.

When you have completed the inventory, sit back and look at it, and ask yourself a number of questions about it.

- What do you think of it yourself?
- Do you have too many cups of tea and coffee?
- What is your sugar intake (remember a lot is hidden in other foods)?
- Do you rely too much on milk products or wheat?
- Do you tend to have cheese too often?
- How much salt do you add and how often?
- How much alcohol do you drink?
- Is there anything you tend to go for rather frequently?
- Do you have chocolate in some form most days?
- How much 'junk' do you eat?
- Do you have enough vegetables and fruit?
- Do you perhaps have too much fruit?
- Do you have too much refined flour products such as white bread, pies, pasta, etc?
- Do your foods contain chemical additives such as colourings, preservatives, flavour enhancers, artificial flavourings, stabilizers, shelf-life enhancers, antioxidants, etc?
- Would you be upset if you were told you ought to stop having a particular item of food or drink for a month or so?
- Is there anything about your diet that is odd in any way or that would be considered at all unusual?
- Remembering the general nutritional advice that is recommended and discussed so widely nowadays in the papers and on television and radio, how does your diet stand up?
- Can you make any improvements?

Some of the questions like 'do you have too many cups of tea or coffee?' are designed to make you look carefully at your diet and ask yourself some honest questions about it. Just about everyone can make some improvements. Most of the other questions require a 'yes' or 'no' answer, although some of them like 'how much salt do you add and how often?' require a different sort of answer. Nevertheless if the answer is basically 'too much' or 'too often', the effect is the same.

On this basis, complete avoidance of a particular item – and I mean *complete* avoidance – is worth trying for a couple of weeks or so, just to see the effect. While your cystitis may not improve in that time, you may find other symptoms benefit, and that will encourage you to keep looking for a dietary cause for your major problems.

If you cut out only one food or drink, when two are implicated, you may not benefit in any obvious way. So, instead of putting that item back into your diet and then avoiding the next one on your list to test, it is best to keep avoiding the first one and then cut number two out as well, and so on. Most of the foods you suspect are not likely to be *essential* to good health, even though they are normally considered healthy foods. For example, while most cheeses are considered good by most nutritionists, with the exception of those with a high salt content like Gorgonzola, you will not become nutritionally deficient without them.

TEA IS AN IRRITANT

The food or drink most commonly associated with chronic cystitis in my experience is tea, which presumably irritates the bladder in some way. It is a more common cause than coffee, so it is likely to be the tannin content rather than the caffeine. On that basis it is worthwhile also avoiding black grapes as they have a high tannin content.

If you avoid something, be careful not to replace it with something else that would take over the problem. If you stop your 10 cups of tea per day for example, don't start having 10 cups of coffee in their place. If you have to drink a lot of fluid with your cystitis, make it bottled or filtered* water wherever possible. Fruit juices should not be taken in large quantities to keep up your fluid intake. Evian water has a high sodium bicarbonate content and can be very useful for that reason.

Many women who develop cystitis regularly, are told to drink as much as possible, without being instructed carefully what to drink. Since tea is 'their drink', it is often the fluid they increase. No one recognizes that the symptoms may actually have got worse as their tea intake has gone up.

The cause and effect are not considered. So the patient goes on the hospital appointment trail which, although it has its value to rule out any obvious anatomical cause, is most commonly of no help to the

**There are various filters on the market at present that fit onto the kitchen tap. Most take out heavy metals such as lead and cadmium, and remove the chlorine. They are not perfect but I recommend improving the water coming from the tap in some way.*

patient, and is extremely costly to the National Health Service.

If you answer the questions on page 125 honestly and set about their correction you will be amazed how your health will improve, and you may even lose your cystitis. The only trouble is you will not know which particular food or drink was responsible for your cystitis or other symptoms. If you want to know, you can always put them back into your diet for a week at a time and see which one or ones reproduce your old symptoms. However, the longer it is since you last ate a food in excess, the less likely it is that symptoms will return even after one week of regularly taking that food.

BEWARE OF WITHDRAWAL SYMPTOMS

If you tidy up your diet all in one go, you could feel much worse for about one week, with a peak of feeling awful around days three and four. If you suddenly stop all tea and coffee, sugar, salt, cheese and junk food at the same time, your body is in for quite a shock. Most of these foods are potentially harmful, although they may not be in any particular person. However, everyone would benefit from reducing them all, and certainly for cutting out all tea, coffee, sugar, added salt and junk. Cheese may be acceptable for some people, but preferably make it the low-salt varieties. If you have a cow's milk allergy, cheese will certainly have to be avoided.

You should, ideally, tidy up your diet and stay on it for about four weeks before abandoning it as of no help. Even if you haven't actually got better for such a change in your eating habits over a month, it is still worthwhile sticking to it. You simply have to look further for a cause for your cystitis.

REINTRODUCING AVOIDED FOODS

When you start adding in first tea, then coffee, sugar, salt, cheese, junk foods, etc., having improved for avoiding them all, if you add in each item of food for approximately one week, it will take at least five weeks before you introduce cheese or six weeks for junk foods. So you will have avoided each for nine and 10 weeks respectively. This avoidance gap may be sufficiently long for your body to have thrown off its reaction to that food. You may therefore not feel unwell during the week of introduction. If you deduce from this that your recovery was merely a coincidence, and start eating all these undesirable foods again, you are likely to go gradually downhill again.

The purpose of reintroducing the avoided foods if you definitely felt better without them is to try to find which ones in particular make you feel unwell. If your taking them makes you feel unwell only when you reintroduce coffee for example, it will be wise to avoid coffee in the main for the rest of your life.

If you don't react to tea, salt, cheese, sugar or junk foods on reintroducing them back into you diet, it would still be wise to avoid them wherever possible, but you will now know that coffee is the main culprit, and that having the others occasionally will not do any harm. In fact, if you avoid coffee for three months, the odd cup will most likely not do any harm either.

The principle behind this avoidance and introduction pattern is that the longer you avoid anything, the less likely you are to react the next time you are exposed to it. If, however, after a period of avoidance you start taking that food again, you can resurrect your allergy to it again, although on rare occasions the avoidance seems to settle it forever.

An example of what can happen with allergies is hay fever. When the grass pollen season comes to an end around August or September, a person's hay fever symptoms gradually settle and disappear, and the patient remains symptom-free until spring of the following year. In mid-May or thereabouts the grass pollen count in the atmosphere gradually rises, but a hay fever sufferer may be exposed daily to increasing levels of grass pollen for two weeks or more before his symptoms start to re-appear, because he has been free of exposure to grass pollen from August to May, which is nine months.

This simple approach to your diet may be all you need, and whether you bother with challenge experiments or not is entirely up to you. If you go on to the new diet for three months or more before allowing yourself to stray a little, feeling well is all that really matters. It is not important to identify the previous main culprit. All the changes you have made are for the good, and your nutritional status will be greatly improved. You will catch colds far less easily, you will feel generally better and more energetic, and your family and friends will tell you how much better you look.

If you were previously overweight, you should lose half to one stone in the first month, and more will come off gradually over the next few months, although you may need to build up some sort of exercises to get yourself into good shape once again. It is best to obtain professional advice about this. Don't just start exercising vigorously. It will do more harm than good.

Most of the items now being avoided need not be replaced with anything in particular. Sugar and salt can simply be avoided. Cheese can be left off salads, or tomatoes put on toast instead of cheese. Cottage cheese may be quite acceptable if milk is not a problem. Junk foods should be replaced by natural foods prepared at home from the basic ingredients.

Breakfast can be muesli (with fruit juice for the milk-allergic or goat's or soya milk as substitutes), or start the day with half a grapefruit or a compote of fruits, or occasionally bacon and eggs (again beware of salt in most bacons). A salad will do for lunch. Cold meat, fish or meat with two vegetables and (low salt) gravy will do for the two main meals. Mid-meal snacks (which you will soon find you don't need anyway) can consist of fruit, nuts, carrots, sticks of celery, pieces of cauliflower, sunflower or pumpkin seeds. There really is a very wide choice nowadays so there should be no excuses for laziness.

CHARTING FOOD PREFERENCES

An alternative way of looking at your diet, or more sensibly one done in conjunction with the four or seven day inventory, is to compile a chart of your likes and dislikes. Table 9.3 gives a shortened version of what I mean, and should be expanded to include absolutely everything you put into your mouth.

9·3 FOOD PREFERENCES

	A	B	C	D	E	F	G
Cup of tea						●	
Cup of coffee					●		
Sugar					●		
Milk				●			
Orange juice				●			
Orange squash			●				
Whole orange				●			
Bread				●			
Butter				●			
Cake				●			
Beef			●				
Bacon		●					
Egg			●				
Potatoes			●				
Cabbage			●				
Carrots			●				
Broccoli		●					
Rice			●				
Salt					●		
Chocolate							●
(continue the list on)							

A *I dislike it or it gives me some symptoms such as indigestion or headache.* **B** *I am not too fond ot it.* **C** *I can take it or leave it.* **D** *I am rather fond of it.* **E** *I am very partial to it.* **F** *I must have it regularly, probably every day, and likely more than once. I would be upset if I was told I must stop having it.* **G** *I definitely crave it.*

Patients often tell me that, if they have *too much* coffee, for example, it can give them a headache. Any symptoms you associate with a food, whether it is taken in small or large amounts, should be ticked in column A. Your body is trying to tell you something which you are ignoring at your peril. Once you have avoided that food deliberately for about three weeks, having it occasionally after that should do you no harm.

I commonly find patients have the information with which to alleviate their symptoms, but they simply have not put two and two together. A professor recently asked me to help him with his psoriasis and gout. When I asked him about any foods he thought might aggravate or cause his symptoms, he said that his last bad attack of gout had occurred when he was examining students in the summer. The university had naturally entertained him to dinner the evening before, and the next day his foot was very inflamed and painful, and he had to do his examining in considerable discomfort. He suspected the double helping of strawberries the night before!

When I asked him what jams he ate, he said his wife was particularly good at making strawberry and raspberry jam to which he was quite partial, and which he ate regularly. His latest minor attack coincided with the opening of a new jar, and his admitted slight overindulgence at the weekend. Avoidance and challenge proved the point. He had simply missed the obvious connection, despite his reasonable suspicions. I am totally convinced that there *is* an explanation for all symptoms and diseases. It is simply a matter of finding it. This applies to chronic cystitis as much as any other condition.

Columns B, C and D are the sort of average response to most foods. We all have our likes and dislikes, and there is nothing wrong with that. No two people look alike so why should our tastes be the same? It's when there is some attitude to a food or drink that is outside a reasonable 'norm' that suspicion should be aroused.

Column E – 'I am rather partial to it' – should be considered with suspicion. It is important to think clearly what the food means to you, and perhaps more importantly how often you eat it. Personally I am very partial to Chinese food or curries, but I only eat either of them once a month or even less frequently, and when I do I am not aware that they harm me. If they did I would most likely be aware of it and hence would try to find out what ingredient was responsible.

When it comes to an unreasonable liking for something, I have allowed two gradings, F and G. People don't often admit to craving something, certainly not a food. They may acknowledge a craving for chocolates, something sweet, or tea or coffee. While their attitude to milk, cheese or bread, as examples, may in fact be a craving, they are more likely to put a tick in Column F than Column G.

Now you have assessed your preference rating for each item of your diet, set about avoiding all those ticked in columns A, F and G, the extremes of the range. Remember withdrawal symptoms in the first week or so, after which your health should begin to improve, and hopefully your cystitis will go away, never to return, unless you slip up on your diet. Again, remember that if you avoid those foods strictly for about three months, having them again occasionally after that should not lead to symptoms. If you think you have been 'cured' by three months of avoidance, your symptoms are likely to return if you over-indulge again at any time in a food you previously established was causing your symptoms.

Using these methods of assessing a diet are not the answer to everyone's problems. When I think back at some of the foods I eventually decided were causing some of my symptoms, I had no particularly unusual attitude to milk. I would probably have put it in column C or possibly column D, although at the time I might have acknowledged that to avoid it would be inconvenient rather than anything else.

I probably developed an allergy to corn (maize) as a result of eating far too many plates of cornflakes, with lashing of sugar and the top of the milk, when I was a student. I loved it, yet never craved it, nor had withdrawal symptoms when I eventually stopped it. I would have put it in column E – 'very partial to it'. As I have said, column E is a suspicious one. If your symptoms have not settled for avoiding foods in columns A, F and G, eliminate those in column E and see what happens. If there is no change in four weeks it is unlikely that this approach will help you find the answer. On rare occasions I have originally tested someone and found only one food, usually milk, producing a positive reaction. On avoiding it for one month, there was no improvement. In fact it took three months for symptoms to clear. The patient I can remember best had rheumatoid arthritis. Presumably his joints needed time to get the fire out of them.

THE FIVE DAY FAST

The five day fast is considered by many clinical ecologists to be an essential part of the treatment of a patient with ecological illness. While some patients' symptoms may be induced primarily by environmental allergies, such as North Sea Gas, house dust, car exhaust fumes, etc., it is unusual for these substances to be part of an addictive stage three reaction. In general, avoidance of chemical allergens leads to a rapid improvement in health. Having said that, I have known a painter and decorator seek out the smell of fresh paint while on holiday, and a petrol pump attendant spend as much time as possible at a petrol station.

Nearly all patients have food and environmental allergies, even if some of them are not very important. However, by the time severe symptoms have developed, one or more foods will be producing addictive symptoms, and it may be essential to break the addictive pattern before a significant improvement is made. To test a person's reaction to a food when the whole body is suffering from addiction may well result in failure to prove that the food is causing symptoms. The addictive pattern is broken by the five day fast.

9·4 FIVE-DAY FAST (BLANK)

Year	*0 = none* 1 = *very mild* 2 = *mild* 3 = *moderate* 4 = *severe* 5 = *very severe*								
Date	SYMPTOMS								Weight
Take Epsom Salts this morning									

The Five Day Fast is exactly what its title suggests – five whole days of spring or bottled water only. Absolutely nothing else must be taken by mouth. The fast must be planned adequately in advance and notes made of progress, good or bad. Table 9.4 shows an example of a blank form that can be used, in which there are nine days of a run-in period, when you eat and drink as usual, without avoiding anything special. It is not necessary to have nine days charted before you start the fast. Five days will do. Weigh yourself first thing every morning, having been to the toilet to empty your bladder, and bowels if possible, standing on the scales completely naked. It does not matter if the scales are inaccurate, so long as they are consistent and the same ones are used each day.

Fill in the top of each column with any symptoms you regularly suffer from, using a point scoring system (0=none, 1=very mild, 2=mild, 3=moderate, 4=moderately severe, 5=severe) for each symptom according to your own interpretation of how bad each one has been in the past 24 hours. This is very much a subjective assessment, and at times it will be difficult to decide on a grade. For example, a headache may be excruciating for 10 to 15 minutes only on one day but merely annoying for 24 hours on another day. In that case, the latter will go down as, say, grade 2, with the former as grade 5 (for 15 minutes only), i.e. the time that was very severe will be put down on the paper.

From the morning of day one of the fast for the next complete five days, the only thing you are allowed to take by mouth is as much spring water as you like, preferably at least 1½ litres (about 3 pints), throughout the day. You must take absolutely no food whatsoever and no other form of drink, and definitely no cigarettes.

Certain drugs being taken before the fast begins may present a special problem and should not be stopped without seeking appropriate advice. Many drugs you are taking, however, can probably be stopped without any danger at all, although again you should really ask your doctor or a suitable medical advisor. Drugs such as those used for blood pressure, arthritis, migraine or depression seldom cause serious problems if stopped, except possibly for withdrawal symptoms from tranquillizers. In any case, you probably wouldn't be reading this book if you were better on these drugs. There are, however, a few drugs such as thyroid hormones and corticosteroids which should not be stopped without appropriate advice.

Once you commence the fast, take great care to avoid 'contaminating' your body by mistake. Take the opportunity to buy a new tooth brush, but DO NOT use ordinary toothpaste. Pure sodium bicarbonate and sodium chloride or merely spring water will be quite sufficient for the time being. Most toothpastes have sugar and other ingredients possibly harmful to you. While it is possible to prepare simple meals for the rest of the family, it is best if you avoid seeing or smelling food during the fast, otherwise you make the whole process so much more difficult for yourself. Most cooks lick their fingers during the preparation of food, so you must avoid doing this. Handling flour may allow some to settle on your lips or some to be inhaled. Spray from the peeling of potatoes can enter your eyes, nose, mouth and lungs, and on rare occasions the smell of a food, especially coffee and fish, can induce symptoms. After all, the smell itself is produced by a chemical.

There is now plenty of evidence of the harmful nature of 'secondhand smoke'. Wherever possible, other members of the household should refrain from smoking. Contamination of their clothing may affect you during the fast.

9·5 FIVE-DAY FAST (EXAMPLE)

Year — *0 = none 1 = very mild 2 = mild 3 = moderate 4 = severe 5 = very severe*

Date	SYMPTOMS								Weight
	puffy eyes	itchy eyes	whole body swelling	swollen ankles	headaches	fatigue	mental confusion	'cystitis'	
Fri	4	4	2	2	1	2	0	1	10st.1lb
Sat	3	3	2	2	0	0	0	1	10st.1lb
Sun	2	3	3	2	0	3	0	2	10st.3lb
Mon	3	3	3	3	0	4	0	1	10st.3½lb
Tues	3	2	4½	4½	3	5	0	3	10st.5lb
Wed	3	1	4½	4½	4	5	3	4½	10st.7lb
Thurs	3	1	4	4	4	5	2	4	10st.5lb
Fri	2	0	3	3	0	4	2	4	10st.6lb
Sat	3	1	5	4	1	3	1	3	10st.8lb
Take Epsom Salts this morning									
Sun	5	1	5	5	4	4	2	4½	10st.12lb
Mon	5	1	5	5	5	5	5	4	10st.7lb
Tues	2	1	2	3	1	2	0	1	10st.3lb
Wed	1	0	0	2	0	0	0	0	10st.0lb
Thurs	0	0	0	1	0	0	0	0	9st.12lb

Table 9.5 shows a typical form from a patient who successfully completed the run-in period and the five day fast. On top of the vertical columns are the symptoms she complained of, and the grade she considered she suffered the symptoms on a daily basis. Your chart could look like this, but it might be quite different.

While it may be possible for you to continue working throughout the fast, it is not possible to predict exactly what will happen. You may plan to continue working, but it is important to be so organized that should symptoms become rather severe, it is possible for you to give up everything and fall into bed. The more severe the problems before the fast, the more likely withdrawal symptoms will make it difficult for you to continue working. On the other hand, being on your own may make sticking to the fast all the more difficult. There are certain things it is inadvisable to attempt during the fast, such as driving long distances, any heavy work, or tasks which require important decisions. If you have to travel long distances to see a doctor on day six, if one is taking you through the whole process, you should organize someone else to do most of the driving. It would also be unwise to undertake a journey if there is likely to be heavy traffic.

You may well feel hungry and tired during the fast, so heavy work is not advisable. By all means prune the roses, or do simple tasks, but do not try to shift heavy slabs or push full wheelbarrows. Leave those heavy jobs for another time. It is important to do only simple things and be quite prepared to stop at a moment's notice. Likewise it is not the time to re-wire the house or do some essential plumbing which may not get finished. Jobs requiring important decisions are worthwhile postponing or perhaps the fast should be postponed itself. Withdrawal symptoms may make such decisions very difficult and, if other peoples lives are at risk or something less dramatic is involved, the five day fast is not the time to make those decisions.

WHAT MAY HAPPEN DURING THE FAST

It is worthwhile explaining what may happen to you during a five day fast. Within 24 hours you are likely to have a headache. If you have previously suffered also from headaches as well as cystitis, whether of the migraine or non-migraine type, and especially if you have suffered from them for a long time (making it likely that you are in the addictive stage three), you must expect a severe headache in the early stages of the fast. You may have any treatment provided it does not involve taking drugs. Try a teaspoonful of pure sodium bicarbonate in water. Ice packs, massage, accupressure or acupuncture are acceptable ways of relieving the headache, or simply retiring to bed and sleeping it off. You must not take tablets if possible. Your usual headache-relieving ones may contain cornflour or colouring agents or a whole host of chemicals to which you may be allergic.

You are only likely to feel hungry on the first day, although not everyone does. The greater the degree of hypoglycaemia (low blood sugar) you have previously suffered from, the greater is your hunger likely to be on day one. Often your main problem is forgetting not to eat, since eating has become such a habit. You may have hunger-like stomach pains without the actual sensation of hunger and, of course, Epsom Salts should have their intended action, possibly amounting to frank diarrhoea for a few hours. Certainly the intention of taking the Epsom Salts is to clear out the bowel, which can harbour a considerable amount of residue from foods.

On the first day of the fast, you may feel dizzy and lightheaded, especially on getting up from the floor or a chair too quickly. While you may not feel too hungry, you may develop an intense craving for certain foods, particularly something sweet like chocolate, but it can often be for something savoury like cheese. Your craving may be for a particular food or combination of foods such as pie and chips. Women in particular crave a cup of tea, although the desire may not be so much a craving as a habit.

Symptoms of a more vague nature, such as aches and pains, moodiness or depression, fatigue, loss of concentration, may gradually get worse during day two to reach a peak on the third day. While these symptoms may reach a peak on day two or days four or five, they are most commonly reached on day three. At the same time more specific symptoms such as palpitations, a general headache, backache, sweating and nausea, will tend to be at their worst on day three.

On the morning of day four, you should wake up feeling very much better. If you suddenly find that any withdrawal symptom previously recorded as severe or worse is now moderate or even mild, by day five it may well have settled completely. The speed with which the symptoms subside after reaching their peak on day three is quite remarkable and can be most gratifying. You may well comment on how good it is to feel so well, saying 'I cannot remember when I last felt as good as this' or 'I had forgotten what it was like to feel so well.'

Most patients follow this pattern, but some of you will range on either side, either reaching a peak of withdrawal symptoms earlier, so feeling well during the fast longer, or peak more slowly, only just beginning to improve by the morning of day six. On occasions, it would be valuable to extend the fast beyond five days, but this is only realistic when you are being monitored as an in-patient in a hospital ward or clinic. In that case the fast can be shortened or extended as needed. If you fast on your own, however, five days is the ideal length and, even if your symptoms haven't subsided properly, you can commence the next phase, of reintroducing foods one by one, on the morning of day six.

The amount of weight you may lose during the fast varies according to your condition prior to commencing it. If your symptoms were moderate to severe in the run-in period, the total weight you will lose during the fast will be more than if the symptoms during the run-in period were only mild. If in fact you do not have food allergies, you should lose approximately 450 g (1 1b) per day on pure spring water only, so that anything in excess of 2.3 kg (5 lb) will be the loss of previously accumulated allergic fluid. As most allergic reactions are accompanied by fluid escaping into the local tissues, the more your allergic reaction the more fluid you will have retained. If you are in a constant allergic state, you will be permanently retaining fluid in your tissues, which you will lose during the fast.

You could easily lose 4.5–6.3 kg (10–14 lb) during the fast, although my record is 9.5 kg (21 lb). If you commence the fast clearly overweight, or are one of those people who have significant fluctuations in weight much of the time, e.g. 3.2 kg (7 lb) up or down in two or three days, your weight loss is likely to be dramatic.

Look at Table 9.5 again. On top of the vertical columns are the symptoms the patient complained of, and the grade she considered she suffered those symptoms on a daily basis. Note the variation in the number of symptoms during the run-in period. The higher the number (indicating greater severity) the heavier she tended to be. During the fast she achieved a very considerable weight loss as the symptoms virtually disappeared all together.

Not all charts will look as perfect as this one and many will show individual variations. Sometimes the grade for fatigue may not appear to have changed at all, but when I ask the patient if the character of her fatigue has changed, she usually gives an emphatic 'yes', indicating that the severe overwhelming fatigue which was previously unrelieved by rest and made her incapable of doing anything, has now been replaced by a relaxed feeling of tiredness, which, however, is not unpleasant. Nevertheless she may still be quite severely fatigued until food is eaten again.

Some clinical ecologists prefer not to fast their patients, but to allow them to eat a handful of foods, often as few as two. By looking at a person's normal diet, two, three or four foods could perhaps be selected that are rarely or infrequently eaten, and so are not likely to be causing the patient's ill health at the time. It will therefore be assumed that she is not allergic to those foods at the start of the period of very restricted eating.

Foods that are found in general to be safe are lamb, round fish (especially the unusual ones like trout rather than cod), pears, broccoli, avocado, although clinical ecologists tend to have their favourites. While it is hoped that these foods are safe, it is not always so. On the other hand, eating only a few foods regularly for five days might induce an allergic reaction to one or more of them, and hence the symptoms will not settle. This is likely to happen in a multiple food-allergic person.

WHO SHOULD AND WHO SHOULD NOT FAST

Remembering that at least 3.2 kg (7 lb) and more may be lost during a five day fast, an overweight person is ideal to undertake it, whereas someone starting somewhat underweight can ill afford a further weight loss. Almost by definition, an overweight person is ill because she is reacting to certain foods by accumulating fluid into her tissues. Fasting and thereby stopping eating those foods will lead to loss of a lot of body fluid. The weight loss is most gratifying.

By contrast, a person who is thin as a result of her food or chemical allergies is not producing her symptoms by accumulation of fluid into the various organs of her body that are complaining. Some other mechanism is involved. Hence a fast is inappropriate.

Another reason why a thin person should not fast is because, by virtue of the chemical mechanisms that produce her symptoms (which we don't fully understand at present), that person tends to be a little more brittle, more ill, and more difficult to get right. She is likely also to have more food allergies than an overweight person and also to have more chemical allergies. During the phase of reintroducing foods, these patients seem to have multiple allergies and to have great difficulty in finding safe foods. This is largely because of the process of unmasking when the range of food allergies is exposed.

The object of a fast or partial fast is to identify foods responsible for a patient's symptoms. At the end of the fast the symptoms should either have cleared or nearly cleared. The patient should certainly be feeling much better at the end of the fast than at the beginning, even if the symptoms became worse to begin with. This makes it possible to identify the former culprits during the phase of reintroducing foods, as on eating certain foods symptoms return. Thus a safe and unsafe list is developed.

REINTRODUCING FOODS

This phase involves the orderly reintroduction of foods one by one to identify those that do and those that do not cause symptoms. It is reasonable to assume that those that do cause symptoms during the second stage were foods previously causing your ill health. Occasionally you may react to a food you rarely eat normally.

As you have just completed a period without food, it is essential to start reintroducing foods that you are not likely to react to. There is no such thing as a totally safe food, i.e. one that no one will react to, but a list can be drawn up of comparatively safe foods, or at least ones that patients do not often react to. Certain clinical ecologists and other practitioners have methods of determining in advance which foods they suspect you might be allergic to, but this will not be gone into here. If safe foods could be anticipated for you, there would be no need to undergo the fast, although it still has obvious advantages, especially for overweight people.

The suggested list of foods and their order of reintroduction should be considered carefully. Such a list is given in Table 9.6. If there are any foods you are already sure upset you, you should not bother to test them. The whole purpose of stage two is to find foods that you *can* now eat safely.

9·6 SUGGESTED FOOD TESTING ORDER

1 Lamb
2 Pineapple
3 Cod
4 Melon
5 Tomato
6 Banana
7 Carrots
8 Whole orange
9 Fresh chicken
10 Peas
11 Beef
12 Olive oil*
13 Cabbage
14 Plaice
15 Onion
16 Tap water
17 Fresh beans
18 Apple
19 Decaffeinated coffee (named brand)
20 Tea
21 Peach
22 Potato
23 Whole egg (not hard boiled)
24 Shredded Wheat
25 ½ glass milk
26 Cane sugar
27 Grapes
28 Pork
29 Mushrooms
30 Rice
31 Cashew nuts
32 Chocolate (dark)
33 Instant coffee
34 White beet sugar

**This will have to be tested with another food, probably cod, banana, fresh chicken or beef.*

If you test immediately after the fast foods you most suspect, your reaction is likely to be severe, as you are in a highly sensitive state at this time. The longer the gap between the last time you ate an unsafe food and the time it is test-eaten, the less severe will be your reaction. On the other hand, if there is any doubt about a particular food, test-eating it after a five day strict avoidance diet will normally clear up whether you are or are not allergic to it.

9·7 FOOD TESTING, PULSE & SYMPTOM CHART

Day	Date	Pulse before	Food being tested	Time food taken	Eaten with	Pulse rate after					Note any reactions that occur and the time they occur
						20 mins	40 mins	60 mins	90 mins	120 mins	

Having selected the foods to be tested in stage two, and the exact order in which you will test them, eat the first food. Take your pulse immediately before and at 20 minute intervals afterwards for one hour, and possibly every half an hour for a further one hour (see Table 9.7). Whenever you take your pulse, you must sit down and rest for five minutes beforehand, so that your body is in a rested steady state. If you do not react to that food within four hours, you may eat the next food. You may only test three foods in any one day, although for some people this rate of reintroduction may be too fast. Some reactions take more than four hours to develop. When you test the first food it obviously has to be taken on its own. When you test the second food, you can eat it with the first food provided it was found to be safe. When you test the third food, you can eat it with the first two foods tested, if you found they were safe. You may test a food, such as plaice or steak, entirely on its own. You don't need to eat other safe foods with it. In fact, it is best if you try to test each food on its own first.

Thus, when testing, you should eat at a sitting a maximum of three foods, i.e. the one you are testing plus any two others you have already found to be safe. You should take each food in the most natural state available and you should not add sauces or spices. Where possible, eat the food raw, as cooking tends to make it less allergenic, although this is not always the case. Cooking rarely makes a food more allergenic. However, I know someone who can eat raw cabbage but gets a very bloated stomach when she eats it cooked. I do not know the explanation for this.

You should avoid tinned food when testing, as various ingredients have usually been added. If fresh peas or beans are not available, for example, choose a well known brand, but before eating them wash them thoroughly in hot water to remove the corn that is often sprayed on them and the E142 which makes them a brighter green for marketing purposes. You should then wash them thoroughly in bottled spring water before you eat them.

If fresh fish is not available, frozen is often quite acceptable. After gutting, fish is usually thrown straight into ice without anything being added. When you test tea and coffee do not add milk, sugar or sweeteners.

REACTION TO A FOOD

Three types of reaction may occur. You will either develop symptoms, a significant *change* in pulse rate or both. Not unnaturally it is the symptoms that are most important. When you take the first food after a five day fast, the gurgling of your intestines getting going again can be ignored, unless you have other symptoms such as pain, diarrhoea or a full feeling.

You should note on a chart any symptoms that occur after testing a food, the time you eat the food and the time symptoms start to reach a peak. Usually an allergenic food will reproduce symptoms you recognize as being those previously causing so much trouble. On occasion, different symptoms can occur. They tend to develop between 15 minutes and three to four hours after eating the food, but the reaction can take in excess of four hours to develop. If this becomes obvious, the interval between testing one food and the next should be lengthened. Some foods take more than 12 hours to produce a reaction, and on rare occasions as long as three days. This makes it extremely difficult to identify unsafe ones. Table 9.8 shows the chart completed for the first 12 foods the patient tested. Note the pulse change and development of

9·8 COMPLETED FOOD CHART

Part of food chart completed, showing the reactions that did occur and the time after eating the food.

Day	Date	Pulse before	Food being tested	Time food taken	Eaten with	Pulse rate after					
						20 mins	40 mins	60 mins	90 mins	120 mins	
Fri	2.1.87	83	lamb	1435	—	80	81	80	79	82	No obvious reaction
Fri	2.1.87	82	pineapple	1910	lamb	81	82	81	80	79	"
Sat	3.1.87	78	cod	0800	pineapple	80	78	79	78	79	"
Sat	3.1.87	79	melon	1230	cod	78	79	78	80	80	"
Sat	3.1.87	77	tomato	1800	lamb melon	77	78	79	77	76	"
Sun	4.1.87	76	banana	0815	cod	77	76	77	76	78	"
Sun	4.1.87	78	carrot	1300	lamb pineapple	79	78	77	78	76	"
Sun	4.1.87	76	chicken	1745	tomato melon	80	88	94	90	80	Stomach started to swell at about 1900 hrs. Stomach pains began at 2100 hrs., continuing all night. Swollen ankles in the morning, passed urine twice during the night. Weight went up 5lb. It took 2 days to return to normal. Felt pretty awful for 24 hrs.
Tues	6.1.87	77	peas	0930	cod	76	75	77	78	77	No obvious reaction
Wed	7.1.87	75	tea	0945	melon pineapple	85	90	96	92	83	Stomach started to swell within 2½ hrs. By 4 hrs quite severe lower abdominal discomfort, with obvious cystitis. Passed urine 10 times in 24 hrs!!
Fri	9.1.87	72	beef	1300	tomato	71	72	73	72	71	"
Sun	11.1.87	69	cabbage	1315	beef tomato	70	71	70	72	71	"
Wed	14.1.87	65	frozen green beans	1930	lamb	66	65	67	68	66	"

symptoms of cystitis after a cup of tea, and the swelling and pulse change that took place after she ate chicken. All the others on this chart were completely clear of a pulse change or symptoms, although they had others later on.

TESTING THE PULSE

The first sign that symptoms of cystitis may soon develop after eating a food is a change in pulse rate, the change usually being upwards, although it may fall. If you eat a reasonable amount of food at a meal, an increase in your pulse rate is a normal physiological reaction to aid digestion. If you take sensible quantities when testing, there should hardly be any change in pulse rate if you are not allergic to any of the foods being tested.

The pulse rate change that may indicate that you have just taken an allergenic food is usually in excess of 10 beats per minute, although there is nothing sacrosanct about this degree of change. A typical reaction will show, say, a 10 to 15 beats per minute rise in 20 minutes, and a further 10 to 15 rise at 40 minutes, either going higher at 60 minutes and levelling off, or coming down. If your pulse rate changes to this extent, you are likely to have symptoms some time afterwards, remembering that the effect on your bladder to cause cystitis can be via the blood stream and not necessarily via the urine.

As symptoms may occur without a significant change in your pulse rate, minor changes may well occur without your realizing their significance. On the other hand, if you eat two or more foods together subsequently, each one of which when tested only produced a small change in pulse rate without any symptoms, they might produce symptoms when you eat them together.

Another reason for taking note of any early changes in pulse rate is because symptoms may be delayed. A significant pulse rate change is nearly always indicative that symptoms are not far behind. In that case, you should start taking steps to minimize the reaction that is likely to follow.

If your symptoms clear well by the end of the fast, especially if withdrawal symptoms occurred at the beginning, sooner or later a food *will* produce symptoms during the stages of testing. All you need is a demonstration of cause and effect. There is no need for symptoms to be severe for you to have that proof. So once symptoms have begun or there has been a significant change in pulse rate, you should begin to lessen the impact.

TURNING OFF A REACTION

Put one teaspoonful of potassium bicarbonate and two teaspoonsful of sodium bicarbonate into half a tumbler of warm spring water. Stir until dissolved, and drink it. This mixture may taste horrible, so a second glass, containing spring water only, should be available to rinse out your mouth. If the taste of this amount of sodium and potassium bicarbonate is too strong, you may dilute it further with spring water. It does not matter how much liquid you take. What is important is the total amount of each powder. The sodium and potassium bicarbonate should be the B.P. (British Pharmacopoea) variety, which you can obtain from your local chemist.

This mixture is important for two reasons. The first is the laxative (aperient) effect of the potassium bicarbonate. Any of the reacting foods that have not yet been absorbed will be pushed on past the absorptive area of the intestines to the non-absorptive area, so avoiding any more of that food entering the blood stream and so prolonging the effect. Diarrhoea may occur, and this is beneficial, but a sense of 'things moving' may be all you notice. If either occurs, there is no need to take any more potassium bicarbonate. The second value of the mixture is the neutralizing effect of the sodium bicarbonate on the whole body acidity that is always produced when an allergic reaction occurs (this is known as metabolic acidosis).

If the potassium bicarbonate has done its job, a teaspoonful of sodium bicarbonate on its own should be taken hourly or so until the reaction has subsided, and no further testing should be carried out until the symptoms have virtually settled, or certainly until any increase in symptoms can be easily recognized if the next food tested is also a reactive one. If for any reason the reaction to the last food is prolonged, you are still allowed to eat foods that you have already passed as safe.

From about the fifteenth food onwards, you should not test more than two foods per day, as you may need slightly longer to make sure whether a reaction is going to occur or not. Whenever you test a grain, take it on its own. Test wheat by eating Shredded Wheat, the closest it is possible to get to a palatable form of pure wheat, even though there are one or two other ingredients in it. For the exquisitely sensitive individual, Shredded Wheat may not be a suitable test food, but it is for most people. As grains tend to have a slower effect, if you have not had a reaction within the first two hours, take a second helping of grain, approximately the same amount, and monitor your pulse every half an hour for a further two hours. Thus you need four hours when testing grains. If you are suspicious but not sure, go on eating that grain every three to four hours, but don't overdo it.

It is quite common for the grains, especially wheat, to produce symptoms without a change in pulse rate. When you first test them, you may easily miss the symptoms or they may be so mild you ignore them. You may therefore assume that it is safe to continue eating the grains because the test procedure seemed to pass them. If symptoms gradually return without any obvious reason, it is best to stop eating grains. The symptoms usually subside without the development of withdrawal symptoms.

Once you have tested about 30 foods, you should have a good idea whether or not foods are the cause of your previous ill health. It is quite possible, though unusual, for you not to have suffered any symptoms at all after eating any of the foods on this list. Provided that symptoms cleared on the fast after getting temporarily worse and you are still feeling well, you can assume that the food or foods previously causing your symptoms have not yet been tested. Good examples are cheese and white bread.

There are obvious advantages to your developing symptoms after eating a food, if for no other reason than to prove cause and effect. The vast majority of people who are ill and who are being treated by conventional medicine have no idea why they are ill, and can only hope that the treatment prescribed for them works. All too often it doesn't. If you have clear-cut, easily recognizable symptoms after eating one or more foods (especially if your cystitis recurs) following a period of fasting for five days, you at least have an explanation for those symptoms, and have the control of those symptoms within your grasp. If you subsequently eat those foods and cystitis develops, you have only yourself to blame. By avoiding them your cystitis will disappear forever.

THE STONE AGE DIET

One alternative type of diet is known as the Stone Age diet. It involves going on to those foods humans most likely ate around two million years ago, if archaeological studies are to be believed. You should plan the diet properly and let all members of the family know what you are doing and when it will start. Having their co-operation is extremely valuable; if there is only you and your husband at home, and especially if he is somewhat overweight, you might persuade him to try it with you. The Stone Age diet is basically a diet of meat, fruit and clean water, following that most likely to have been eaten by humans in the pre-cereal era of more than forty thousand years ago, with nuts, vegetables and seeds added in. Any food you know upsets you, you should continue to avoid, and possibly also foods in the same biological food family. As an example: potatoes are related to tobacco, tomatoes, peppers (chilli, paprika, green and red peppers) and aubergines. They are all part of the deadly nightshade family.

9·9 THE STONE AGE DIET

	Food allowed
Meat	Lamb, rabbit, venison, hare and any wild meats available. All poultry and game, including chicken, turkey, duck, pheasant, woodcock, partridge and any wild game available. NO beef, veal or pork (including ham and bacon).
Fish	All white fish such as cod, haddock, herring, whiting, plaice, coley and mackerel. Fresh shellfish. Sardines in oil are probably alright. NO smoked or heavily salted fish, fish fingers or fish in batter unless in permitted flours.
Flours	Use potato, pea, buckwheat (not a true grain; it is of the rhubarb family), tapioca, sago and chick pea (Besam gram flour).
Cooking oils	Olive, sunflower, safflower, linseed, almond and apricot kernel oils. DO NOT use 'Vegetable oils' as they are likely to contain corn or soya oils. Use cold-pressed oils if possible.
Nuts	All nuts except peanuts. DO NOT have salted or 'roast' forms. Be safe and crack them yourself.
Fruit	Apples, pears, grapes, pineapples and peaches. NO citrus fruits (oranges, grapefruit, lemons, limes, tangerines, satsumas, clementines) or bananas.
Vegetables and salads	Potatoes, tomatoes, all green leafy vegetables and salad items. NO corn, corn-on-the-cob or sweet corn.
Pulses and seeds	All lentils, beans, pumpkin and sunflower seeds.
Condiments	All herbs, spices and peppers.
Drinks	Bottled water (still or carbonated) or tap water put through a suitable filter. Use it to rinse and cook all vegetables (although they are better eaten raw). Pure chickory, pure dandelion beverages, herbal teas, hot or cold juices of allowed fruits, preferably freshly prepared.

The Stone Age diet allows you to eat a considerable number of foods, but tends to recommend avoiding those foods that have been introduced into human diets in the past few thousand years, and naturally excludes modern foods and all junk foods. It concentrates on natural foods, although it may be very difficult to obtain them nowadays without their having been contaminated by the various chemicals used by farmers. Thus, you may have to compromise.

Foods you can eat are given in Table 9.9. The list includes some meats but not all. The reason beef and pork are excluded is because they have become so heavily polluted by hormones. The safer meats,

9·10 THE STONE AGE DIET

	Foods to avoid
Grains	Barley, corn (maize), millet, oats, rice, rye, sugar cane, wheat. Avoiding these means many of the staple items of your diet, such as bread, biscuits, cakes, gravy mixes, pastries, pies, spaghetti, pasta, soups, jams, thickeners and sauces.
Meat	No beef, veal or pig meat.
Dairy products	Eggs, milk, cheese, butter, yoghurt (whether from cow's, goat's or sheep's milk).
Certain fruits	Bananas and all citrus fruits (oranges, lemons, limes, grapefruits, tangerines, clementines, satsumas and mandarines).
Yeast products	No Marmite, Bovril, Oxo and other gravy mixes. No vinegar. No mushrooms or alcohol or any sort. No cheeses or fermented drinks.
Drinks	No tea, coffee, or alcohol. No sugary pop such as Coca Cola, 7 Up or squashes that have sugar or colourings or other additives.
Additives	No colourings, food additives, flavourings, preservatives.
Sugar	No sugar in any form whether cane or beet. No chocolate, sweets or candies.
Soya	No soya products, whether put into foods or of a purer form such as soya milk.
Junk food & mixtures	As all the foods on the allowed list are in their natural state, foods prepared by the food industry, especially anything in a packet, should be avoided. If in doubt, leave it out.
Vitamins & minerals	These should not be taken during the Stone Age diet. Your better diet should make them unnecessary.
Medication	This prevents a lot of problems. If they are not really helping you they can probably be stopped, but it would be unwise to do without them without first checking with your doctor whether they are 'essential' or not. Unfortunately, many of them contain things such as corn starch, lactose (milk sugar) or colourings.

and wild game, are included. Fresh fish is allowed but not smoked fish, shell fish or fish in batter, unless made from ingredients that are on your allowed list. Most vegetables are allowed but not soya, which is a comparatively recent addition to man's diet. As citrus fruits seem to be high on most clinical ecologists' list of unsafe foods in cystitis, they should be avoided. Certain modern oils like sunflower and safflower seem to be safe. Most nuts, fruits and seeds are on the safe list, but not all of them.

Table 9.10 gives the foods that should be avoided. It includes ALL grains (including rice), all diary products (eggs, milk, cheese, butter, yoghurt and foods made from cow's milk), all additives, sugar, tea, coffee and yeast-based foods. Although the list of what not to eat is comprehensive, there is a lot left to eat, but you will need to plan ahead and make sure you have certain items of food in stock. You would also be wise to seek out suppliers whose products you can be sure of.

While you ought to avoid grains, it may be safe to eat free-range chickens that have been fed on grain. Soya-fed chickens are unwise, but may be acceptable to your particular metabolism. Obtain organically-grown vegetables where possible. Seek out allotment-keepers who have spare produce but ask what sort of manure, fertilizers and chemicals they have used before you buy anything.

As far as drinks are concerned, pure water is ideal, but certain herbal teas and chicory are considered acceptable. To begin with you may not like them, but it is amazing how quickly you become accustomed to them. You may well find this makes you drink far less. If you need to drink a lot to help you get over an attack of cystitis, drink pure water (either bottled spring water or tap water filtered through one of the filters currently available on the market). You are allowed juices from the fruits on your safe list, but they should be freshly prepared from the fruits themselves, if possible. It is, however, becoming more easy to obtain pure fruit juices – the ones in glass bottles are best because most cartons have an aluminium lining.

Although chlorine boils out of water, other chemicals do not. Tap water contains over 100 different chemicals, some of which are beneficial to humans, but the majority are undesirable. Tap water is often re-cycled, so it may contain residues of drugs; other harmful chemicals can also get into the water supply. The pipes leading from the mains in the road to your house may be made of lead, the pipes in your house will certainly be copper, which may dissolve into the water if it is naturally soft and therefore slightly acid. Lead from soldered joints can also get into your drinking water. All of this makes it sensible for you to either drink bottled spring water (which can be sparkling or still), or to filter it at the point of consumption. Use it also to wash and cook your vegetables.

WHAT TO EXPECT FROM THE DIET

The Stone Age diet should be used for a good four weeks. During the first week after you have suddenly avoided a large number of foods you previously took for granted, you must expect withdrawal symptoms. If you feel headachey, light-headed, miserable or bad tempered be assured you are doing yourself good, even though it may be difficult to accept at the time. During the second week things should improve dramatically, although you may suffer somewhat for up to two weeks. Cystitis rarely gets worse as a withdrawal symptom, and is likely to improve.

If you have an addictive pattern of eating before you start the Stone Age diet, you must expect to crave certain foods. Don't loiter in the kitchen. Get up and do something, read a book, go for a walk, play the piano, write the letters that you have been putting off, do anything to stop you thinking about food. As with a fast, it is a good idea to take an adequate dose of Epsom Salts in warm water as you start the diet. You should repeat the dose until you have had a good clear-out of your bowels. It is also sensible to have another clear-out at the beginning of the second week. This should enhance the cleansing of your system.

By the end of four weeks, you should be feeling not only very fit and well, but your symptoms of cystitis should have gone. Many women have a constant feeling that they are about to suffer a major attack; this should disappear and you will come to realize that something you were previously eating was causing the sensation all the time.

9·11 INTRODUCING FOODS

1. Rice
2. Egg
3. Beef
4. Oats
5. Banana
6. Soya
7. Corn (maize)
8. Decaffeinated coffee
9. Grapefruit
10. Barley
11. Goat's milk (you may never have had it before)
12. Millet, tapioca or sago
13. Pork (not ham or bacon)
14. Shredded Wheat
15. A whole orange
16. $1/2$ glass cow's milk
17. Tea

Although there are many other foods, they tend to be mixtures such as bread, cheese or Oxo. In due course, you can try them all unless your experiences so far suggest it is unwise to try some of them. You will note I have left wheat, orange, cow's milk and tea to last, as they are highly suspect. However, I have not even put sugar, colourings or additives on the list at all, as they are best avoided permanently.

REINTRODUCING FOODS

The next step is to introduce back into your diet the foods you have been studiously avoiding for the past four weeks. As you have not had them for a month, you are not lkely to produce obvious reactions when you first eat them. It is important at this stage to make copious notes about what you start eating, when, and how often. If you were to start eating every day a food that was previously responsible for your cystitis or other symptoms, it could take a week or more before the symptoms return. Deciding which of a number of recently reintroduced foods is the culprit can therefore present problems.

Table 9.11 suggests the order in which you can start introducing foods back into your diet. I suggest you only have one food on three days out of seven, and give yourself a rest from eating on every Sunday to begin with, although you may find Sunday a better day to start introducing a new food.

- On days one, three and five of week one have a portion of rice.
- On days two, four and six of week one have an egg.
- On days one, three and five of week two have some beef.
- On days two, four and six of week two have some pure oats (oatcakes or porridge with water or fruit juice).

While the above slow rate of reintroduction may be sensible, it may be perfectly reasonable to have rice and eggs (but at separate meals) on days one, three and five of week one, and beef and oats (also at separate meals) on days two, four and six of week one. In this way you will be introducing four foods in the first week.

The order of foods in Table 9.11 is only a suggestion, but it is based upon my experience of food allergies. I have left wheat, orange, cow's milk and tea to last, as they are highly suspect. However, I have not even put sugar, colourings or additives on the list at all, as they are best avoided permanently. It is by no means ideal for everyone, and each person must select the order for herself. You may decide that a particular food goes with something else to make a new and acceptable meal.

Remember that, if you test at this rate, you will not reintroduce the foods at the end of the list for several weeks. Your lack of a reaction to the last food may suggest that it was not the former culprit. If you therefore start developing cystitis again, you will have to decide which recently introduced foods you are now reacting to.

The ideal way of preventing the re-development of a reaction to a food avoided for many weeks, is to have that food infrequently. If you leave trying tea until the last, however, and no symptoms develop on taking it again, you are likely to slip into your old bad habit of having too many cups every day, so you may re-develop your allergy to tea eventually by having too much of it too often, if it was previously a cause of your cystitis.

When trying to identify food allergies on your own, there is no easy way. All the methods I have described so far need a lot of concentration, effort and time. No method is perfect for every patient, and indeed it may not turn out to be something you are *eating* that is causing your cystitis. It could possibly be a chemical such as North Sea Gas, petrol or diesel fumes, or any one of a number of pollutants you cannot easily avoid. They are also rather difficult to test for, but are fortunately very seldom the main cause of cystitis.

On the other hand, your general health is likely to benefit from some sort of dietary manipulation and you should lose some unwanted weight. Many of the foods you previously consumed in unreasonable amounts you will now avoid, and others you will eat only occasionally. You are likely to think more seriously about what you eat and drink in the future and will hopefully make your family and friends think about their diet, too.

THE ANTI-CANDIDA DIET

If the candida organism is either responsible for or very much a factor in your cystitis, avoiding specific items will starve candida of its natural food. The foods that candida particularly loves are sugar in *all* forms and refined carbohydrate. Milk should also be avoided as it contains a lot of lactose (milk sugar). Because candida is a mould itself, its survival is helped by other foods that are moulds, such as cheese, alcohol, mushrooms, yeast and vinegar.

Table 9.12 lists all the foods that should be avoided strictly if you decide to go onto the anti-candida diet. Ideally you should stay on it for three months, although the very occasional lapse may not matter too much. Try to be *very* strict with yourself, however, for the first four weeks, to give your body a really good chance of starving the candida organisms completely. If you clearly improve on the anti-candida diet, and symptoms return if you stray too early, you will know that it is wise to stick to the diet a month or two longer.

If this degree of dieting is not successful in eradicating candida completely, in contrast to bringing it under control, you would most likely benefit from one of the anti-candida drugs, most of which, however, can only be obtained on prescription. It is likely, also, that there are other factors that must be considered that are contributing to your ill health. I am referring to a high body level of lead, possibly from drinking water, or more likely an allergy to mercury coming from your dental amalgam fillings. This has been publicized a lot recently and I have no doubt whatsoever that it is important in many patients, including those suffering from cystitis. It does NOT affect everyone, so it is important not to have your amalgams replaced with a non-metallic substance without the appropriate advice.

If it is done, the order is important and depends upon the total amount of galvanic current coming from each tooth. I have put this in here not to whet your appetite but to warn you not do something you might later regret, but which you have heard might be important. If you stop a food, you can always start eating it again. Messing about with your teeth can do more harm than good.

It is probably a good idea first, however, to do the four day inventory. Take stock of what you really are eating on a day-to-day basis. Get to know yourself better, your diet, your likes and dislikes. You don't actually need to do the preference list, although it shouldn't take too long and can be quite fascinating to do.

9·12 WHAT TO AVOID ON THE ANTI-CANDIDA DIET

Foods that contain yeast as an additive ingredient: biscuits, breads, pastries, cakes and cake mixes, flour enriched with vitamins from yeast, and meat fried in crumbs.
Foods that contain yeast or yeast-like substances because of their nature or the nature of their manufacture and preparation: mushrooms, cheeses, vinegars such as apple, pear, cider, grape and malt vinegars (although some vinegar is pure chemical acetic acid which could be allowed if you could find some and be sure about it). These vinegars should be avoided in their original state as well as in such foods as mayonnaise, olives, pickles, sauerkraut, horseradish, French dressing and tomato sauce; vitamin products.
Fermented drinks: whisky, gin, wine, brandy, rum, vodka, beer, i.e. *all* alcoholic drinks.
Malted products: cereals, most chocolates and malted milks drinks.
Citrus fruit juices (either frozen or canned): only home squeezed fruit juices are yeast free.
All forms of sugar: white and brown sugar, honey, maple syrup, golden syrup, sweets, toffees, chocolates, candies, ice creams, biscuits, puddings, drinks with added sugar such as squashes, all pop and fizzy drinks including bitter lemon and tonic water.

As so many people crave sugar, when you start on a sugar-free diet, avoid all sugar substitutes.

White flour in all forms: bread, biscuits, puddings, pasta, cakes, which are so heavily refined that yeasts treat them like sugar.

Cow's milk in all forms, because of its lactose (milk-sugar) content, although food combinations containing whey, casiene and albumin *are* allowed.

By listing what you are eating regularly, you can then compare it with the anti-candida diet and see how much you have to change. You are likely to get quite a shock. If your history suggests that candida could be a problem for you, you can see why you are unwell and why a change in your diet could be so important. The chances are you are having far too much sugar, chocolate, cheese and bread.

PLAN THE DIET WELL

It is essential you plan what you are going to do. Remember, as with all forms of diet, that you are likely to feel *worse* to begin with. I described this fully when I explained the Five Day Fast, and it is just as likely to occur when you first cut out too much sugar, chocolates, refined carbohydrate and mould foods.

Withdrawal symptoms must be expected, but fortunately cystitis seldom gets worse. If you do not fast, but choose the anti-candida diet, your withdrawal symptoms may be a little more prolonged, as with the Stone Age diet. Expect them to last up to a week. Strangely, some people might feel better immediately, even though they have been unwell for so long you would expect them to be in stage three of the adaptive mechanisms. I have known a 60-a-day smoker give up cigarettes without a whimper.

If you avoid foods previously causing your cystitis, you may crave those foods during the withdrawal stage, but this is frequently not too much of a problem. When you stop refined carbohydrates to starve candida of its natural food, the organism demands its food and tries to get it from anywhere. As sugar is circulating in your blood, but no longer being pumped into it direct from your diet, candida organisms try to extract the sugar from your blood stream. This tends to make you low in blood sugar for a time, and hence can make you feel hypoglycaemic. However, it is not easy for candida to get sugar from this source, so it tends to be starved of what it would ideally like to have. Persevering with the refined carbohydrate-free diet rather than giving in, ensures that the candida organisms gradually die, but in so doing they may liberate their toxins and make you feel ill. So the first two weeks may be quite a trial for you.

It is important to remember, however, how candida got a hold in the first place. Antibiotics, the contraceptive pill, multiple pregnancies, the wrong diet, all played their part. With any luck your new and improved diet will not only make you more healthy in general terms, making antibiotics less likely in the future, but it will also kill off the candida organisms. You will hopefully never go back on to the contraceptive pill, but whether to embark upon another pregnancy is entirely up to you. If you are feeling better because of your better diet, a new addition to the family could be an added bonus.

It is difficult to tell you how long to maintain the anti-candida diet. It really depends upon how things go for you. If you are simply relying upon a change in your diet to kill off the candida, you will have to stick to it for at least three months, and quite probably much longer, before relaxing it a little. When you do let yourself off the leash don't dive into the sugary foods but rather reintroduce mould-type foods (such as bread, mushrooms and vinegar) first. At the best of times, alcohol should be avoided but I certainly would not want to prohibit it for life. I leave that up to you. However, it would be sensible to avoid sugar, chocolates, and refined white flour in the main for the rest of your life. Where you have control over your eating habits this would be advisable for both you and your family but it could be relaxed when you go out for a meal. Even then you can exercise your prerogative and consciously choose to avoid certain foods. I do.

If you are not feeling much better and your cystitis is still troubling you at the end of a month, the chances are that you are still eating something that should be avoided. This does not mean that the anti-candida diet should be relaxed. It may well be sensible to look at your diet again and consider what action to take. After all, the anti-candida diet doesn't ban tea or coffee, wheat or oranges. You can manipulate your diet further without running into any problems of nutritional deficiencies. You should keep on the anti-candida diet if you originally thought it was appropriate. This way the organism will be brought under proper control.

ADDITIONAL MEASURES TO HELP CONTROL CANDIDA

Nystatin

If adopting the anti-candida diet settles your cystitis and makes you feel better, but you feel unwell when you try to relax the diet a little or your cystitis returns, it suggests that candida has been brought under control but not eradicted. If you are being helped by a clinical ecologist it is possible he will prescribe Nystatin. This is a drug which specifically kills most moulds including candida albicans, and can help you a lot. I am assuming, however, that you are doing all this on your own.

Lactobacillus Acidophilus

As your bowel in particular has been taken over by a colony of candida albicans, the chances are that, even if you bring the numbers of organisms down by denying them their natural food, they are still in greater numbers than any other organisms. They can therefore grow again all too easily if you allow sugar or other refined carbohydrates back into your diet, and this stalemate could continue for ages.

It is, therefore, sensible to replenish your bowel with the normal organisms that were killed off by the antibiotics you had in the past, that have now been replaced by a colony of candida albicans. Lactobacillus acidophilus in pure culture form is obtainable from various suppliers. The dosage varies somewhat according to the origin and form, but many billions of organisms (usually a quarter to one teaspoonful) should be taken daily. It may also be worthwhile putting some in your vagina at night if you definitely have thrush or an unexplained discharge.

Biotin

Tablets of Biotin 500mcg could be beneficial. They can be obtained from your local health food store or direct from a supplier. They are rather expensive as the dose should ideally be two tablets three times daily, although half that dose may be enough, and will certainly help.

Caprylic Acid

The normal bowel organisms and break-down products of digestion produce many chemicals, among them the short-chain fatty acids. These acids exert a natural control over unwanted yeasts, fungi and other organisms, and are part of the way the healthy bowel keeps itself in a good condition.

Part of your treatment to help eradicate rather than simply control candida albicans could be taking doses of fatty acids by mouth, the most effective of which is caprylic acid. While it has been known for some time to be effective against pathogenic organisms in the laboratory and experimental animals, its main drawback has been that it is destroyed by the processes of digestion if taken by mouth. Recently, however, tablets of caprylic acid have been formulated that get round this particular problem.

As caprylic acid is not a drug but a nutritional way of treating candida, it does not need a prescription, although it can be prescribed on the NHS if a doctor is willing to oblige. Unfortunately, it is not readily available in the United Kingdom.

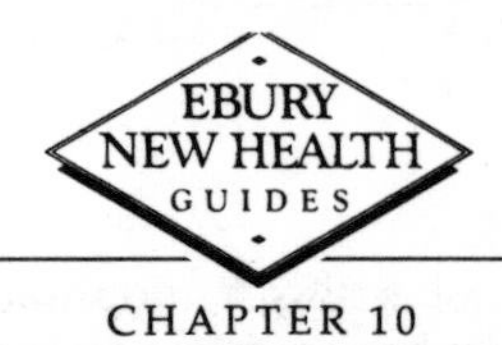

CHAPTER 10

HOW TO DEAL WITH AN ATTACK OF CYSTITIS

THE whole of this book so far has told you how to prevent the next attack and how to track down the basic cause of your cystitis. Before you decide which diet to adopt, and indeed when you reintroduce foods you temporarily avoided, you may well have an attack of cystitis. It is all very well my telling you how to fiddle with your diet, but it will take some weeks to sort it all out, so you need to know how to deal with any attack that occurs in the meantime.

Prepare yourself by buying from your local chemist a bottle of dip-stick papers for testing your urine. These will help establish whether your urine is acid (pH 1–7), which it is likely to be, or alkaline (pH 7–14). They will also identify the presence of protein. Protein in the urine will suggest that you have an infection, but it does not prove it. Remember, antibiotics have not helped in the past, so there is no need to rush off to your doctor.

If you are having a food allergy reaction, your whole body will tend to become slightly acid (as a result of the release of acidic chemicals from your cells) which the body doesn't like. You are designed to be just on the alkaline side (pH of about 7.4), so to rid your body of this extra acid, your kidneys excrete it, thus making your urine acid. On rare occasions, a genuine infection is caused by certain organisms such as proteus, which split urea to liberate ammonia. Not only will your urine turn the test paper alkaline but in such cases, it will also have a strong smell of ammonia.

KEEP YOUR FLUID LEVELS UP

As there is always the possibility that an infection is involved (though it is seldom the real cause), you must flush your bladder out. Just about everyone knows this, and you would be wise to stick to either filtered or pure bottled spring water. Take a sample of your urine as soon as your feel the first signs of an impending attack of cystitis and test it for pH and protein. Drink 600 ml (1 pint) of water straightaway and then at least 300 ml (1/2 pint) every hour for the next four hours, by which time you will have drunk 1.5 litres (3 pints). Thereafter, keep your fluid intake up but not at such a high level. With any luck you will already be feeling better, or certainly confident that you have contained the worst of it. If this is the case you can reduce the volume to 300 ml (1/2 pint) every two to three hours for the next eight hours. For the next two to three days, drink 1.8–2.4 litres (3–4 pints) in 24 hours.

MAKE YOUR URINE ALKALINE

When I looked up a clinical pharmacology book dated 1966, to see what was being advised then, there was the usual advice about the antibiotics available at the time. There was also some most interesting information which today's doctors would rarely take into account, but which is still appropriate, all the more so if my approach to recurrent cystitis is considered.

12·1 FLUID INTAKE

	At onset of symptoms	+ 1 hour	+ 1 hour	+ 1 hour	+ 1 hour	+ 2 to 3 hours	+ 2 to 3 hours	+ 2 to 3 hours	+ 2 to 3 hours	
Actual time										*For the next 12 to 24 hrs adjust your fluid and sodium bicarbonate intake according to results.*
pH of urine										
Drink pure water	1 pint	1/2 pint	1/2 pint	1/2 pint	1/2 pint	1/2 pint	1/2 pint	1/2 pint	1/2 pint	
Amount of sodium bicarbonate added	flat tsp.	flat tsp.	flat tsp.	flat tsp.	flat tsp.	1/2 – 1 tsp.	1/2 – 1 tsp.	1/2 – 1 tsp.	1/2 – 1 tsp.	
						(depending upon pH of urine)				

The first fact I noticed was the statement that dysuria (the pain of passing urine) is relieved by altering urinary pH from acid to alkaline. If it has been established, why on earth don't doctors recommend it? Are they so blinded by the science of antibiotics that they are not concerned about their patients' discomfort? One method the book recommends to make your urine alkaline is 3 g of sodium bicarbonate (approximately a level teaspoonful of pure B.P. powder) in water by mouth every two hours until the pH of your urine is 7.0 or above. The dose should then be adjusted to keep it there. As you will be drinking a lot of fluid anyway, you could add sodium bicarbonate each time. If you follow the advice detailed in Table 12.1 you should take in enough yet not overload your system. Write yourself out a chart as in the table, and pin it up somewhere. This will have the added bonus that you will feel that you are doing something positive to help yourself.

As soon as you feel the first signs of cystitis developing, pass a sample of urine and measure its pH. Write it down on the chart. Drink 600 ml (1 pint) of slightly warmed water containing about a flat teaspoonful of pure sodium bicarbonate (put powder into a teaspoon and flatten it off with a knife). This should then weigh about 3 g ($^{1}/_{4}$ oz). This quantity of sodium bicarbonate in a whole pint does not taste at all unpleasant, but you can always rinse your mouth out afterwards if you want to.

Every time you pass urine from now on until the attack has cleared or not fully developed, test the pH of your urine and note it on the chart. Table 12.2 shows what your own chart could look like. Within 12 hours of following this regime your symptoms should have gone, but it is sensible to keep your fluid intake much higher than normal for the next 24 hours or so.

12·2 EXAMPLE OF FLUID INTAKE CHART DURING AN ATTACK OF CYSTITIS

	At onset of symptoms	+ 1 hour	+ 1 hour	+ 1 hour	+ 1 hour	+ 2 to 3 hours	+ 2 to 3 hours	+ 2 to 3 hours	+ 2 to 3 hours	
Actual time	7.00pm	8.00pm	9.00pm	10.00pm	11.00pm	mid-night	1.00am	2.00am	3.00am	*For the next 12 to 24 hrs adjust your fluid and sodium bicarbonate intake according to results.*
pH of urine	6.0	6.0	6.5	6.75	7.00	7.00	7.00	7.25	7.50	
Drink pure water	1 pint	1/2 pint	1/2 pint	1/2 pint	1/2 pint	1/2 pint	1/2 pint	1/2 pint	1/2 pint	
Amount of sodium bicarbonate added	flat tsp.	flat tsp.	flat tsp.	flat tsp.	flat tsp.	1/2 – 1 tsp.	1/2 – 1 tsp.	1/2 – 1 tsp.	1/2 – 1 tsp.	
						(depending upon pH of urine)				

The other way you can acidify your urine is to take potassium citrate mixture BPC which you could buy from your chemist, and keep in a cupboard at home ready for instant use. The mixture is made up to contain 3 g of potassium citrate in 10 ml (two teaspoonfuls), and you should take two to four teaspoonfuls every six hours, which can be put into the water you will also be drinking. This standard preparation contains citric acid so just might make you worse if citrus fruits are a cause of your cystitis. Potassium citrate can, unfortunately, also cause a sense of nausea.

The old clinical pharmacology book also said that an alkaline urine not only makes many of the standard antibiotics more effective, but that it discourages the growth of *E. coli*. You may remember that I said *E. coli* is the most common organism involved in cystitis, so making the urine alkaline makes good sense.

Although tetracycline is not often used nowadays for cystitis, it works better in an acid urine, while sulphonamides (which are still used a lot) work better in an alkaline urine.

A word of caution here. Many people take ascorbic acid (vitamin C) whenever they think they have an infection. It is sensible not to use it in cystitis, and to stop it temporarily if you are taking it when an attack begins as it makes urine very acid. If you must take vitamin C take the sodium ascorbate form.

Because sodium bicarbonate can be so effective if taken at the first signs of an impending attack of cystitis, you would be wise to carry in your handbag enough powder for the first 12 hours of treatment. Put about five flat teaspoonfuls of powder into a suitably sized tablet bottle, which I am sure your local chemist will willingly supply for you. The smallest bottle (15 g (1/2 oz) tablet bottle) will hold three teaspoonsful, enough for the first four hours.

If you are going on a car journey, especially over a weekend when it may be difficult to find a chemist open, put 1.2 litres (2 pints) of spring water into a bottle together with two flat teaspoonfuls of sodium bicarbonate. This will give you enough for the first two hours anyway. You can also carry some extra powder for use when you reach your destination, or find a hotel or restaurant that is obliging. Incidentally, Evian water contains sodium bicarbonate so it is a most suitable bottled water to have in the house, although the amount it contains is not high.

USE A HOT WATER BOTTLE

If you are at home when an attack starts, and you do not succeed in controlling it quickly using a lot of liquid plus sodium bicarbonate, place a hot water bottle between your legs. It should be a comfortable temperature, and should certainly not burn you. Put a clean cotton towel between the hot water bottle and your vaginal area. Replenish the bottle every so often to keep it comfortably warm.

USE WITCH-HAZEL SOAKS

Every so often, soak some clean non-coloured cotton wool in witch-hazel and apply it to your urethral opening. In some people this can have a most soothing effect, and of course the use of witch-hazel is a time-honoured treatment for cuts and bruises, helping to keep them clean and free from infection.

BATHE

At the onset of an attack of cystitis, sitting in a comfortably hot bath swooshing water between your legs can be quite soothing. Don't forget to dry yourself with a clean *white* towel.

There are one or two practical tips that are worth following if you suffer regular attacks of cystitis.

Underwear

Always use cotton underwear and try to avoid nylon and similar materials and also try to avoid wearing tights. Because they do not 'breathe' so well, they encourage a warm, moist environment around your vaginal area (which tends to be this way inclined anyway), which will encourage the growth of candida if it is already a problem. If you must wear tights, make sure your underwear is cotton. You might be willing to go back to stockings and a suspender belt; it all depends upon fashions of the day. You can buy elasticated stockings.

Trousers

For the same reason as above, avoid wearing trousers, unless they are comfortably loose between your legs. I am not expecting you to look a mess, however. Again, if you must wear trousers, choose a cotton pair if possible.

Skirts

Skirts and dresses are ideal, but culotte skirts should be avoided although they are rarely designed to reach high into the crutch. Try to avoid man-made fabrics even in your skirts and dresses. You will be sitting down much of the time so the material will mould itself into your lap and prevent a free flow of air between your legs.

No underwear

If you are daring enough, the weather is not cold, your outfit is appropriate, and you are not going to do any bending, try not wearing underwear at all.

Soap

Never use soap to wash the vaginal area. You don't wash your eyes out in soap, so why insult your other delicate tissues with it. Avoid all 'bath salts' when bathing as they, too, can be an irritant.

Lavatory Paper

A soreness in the vaginal or urethral area can be caused by using *coloured* lavatory paper after going to the toilet. I can remember two women in whom this was a major contributory cause. Other patients had already gone back to white tissues without any improvement in their cystitis, as they also had food allergies and candida. It was therefore not possible to know how important the colourings might have been.

On rare occasions, though I have not met it myself but it is worth mentioning here, formalin used in some tissues to make them softer could be a cause of cystitis. I have read of such cases being reported from America. If there is any question this could be important, dry between your legs with a warm air dryer. If you use a towel, the detergents might be just as much of an irritant in an extreme situation.

Hygiene

When a harmful organism is cultured in the urine of a sufferer from cystitis, it is most commonly *E.coli*, although there are others. *E.coli* is a common inhabitant of the bowel, so the bowel in such a person could be a reservoir for this organism. While it is just feasible that these organisms might spread from the rectum forwards to the urethra, somehow skirting round the vaginal opening, it is more likely to get there if you wipe yourself, after opening your bowels, from the back forwards. You should therefore *always* wipe from in front backwards.

Cystitis and Sexual Intercourse

While it is possible for unusually frequent intercourse, possibly accompanied by too much alcohol, to precipitate a particular attack of cystitis, many women are aware that an attack can occur at any time. I have tried to explain that if you follow the advice I have given, the *underlying* reason why you are more prone to cystitis after intercourse will be eliminated. Nevertheless it is sensible to use any means possible to reduce the likelihood that sexual intercouse will once again leave you suffering. Never have intercourse on a full bladder, and, as soon after intercourse as possible, go to the toilet and pass water. Any germs that might possibly be forced into the bladder by the act of intercourse will be washed out immediately. While you may not feel like getting out of bed at this particular time, this simple trick could save you a lot of discomfort.

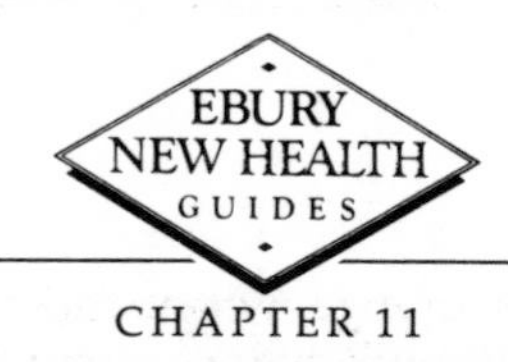

CHAPTER 11

PLANNING YOUR OWN CURE

I HOPE you are now convinced that, if you do something about your diet, you really could soon be rid of cystitis. I and my colleagues who practice clinical ecology and nutritional medicine have helped so many women that we certainly have no doubt that your cystitis can be cured.

In this chapter I want to give a thumbnail sketch of how to set about changing your diet for the better. The last chapter described five different methods you can use, but to a certain extent they can be combined. Ideally, you should find a doctor or other practitioner who can guide you, whose methods might cut a few corners.

PHASE 1

Before you *change* your diet, you really must find out *what* you are eating. It is no good guessing. You must write it down, not a day or so later but as you eat it.

Do the four or seven day inventory (page 81), and do it properly. Don't cheat. Write down *everything* you put into your mouth for at least four days, trying not to change your regular eating habits. Then sit back and look at the chart and answer all the questions listed on page 125. It is distinctly possible that the clue to your cystitis will be in these questions. Because embarking on a change of diet can obviously present you with certain problems, it really would be worth doing the food preference rating, so that you will hopefully get it right from the start.

PHASE 2

The next stage is to try to decide if you have a candida problem or if a particular food is causing your cystitis. I would say that candida is an important cause in 80 per cent of people suffering from recurrent or chronic cystitis. In the remaining 20 per cent, and in at least 30 per cent of those in whom candida is a major cause, foods not on the anti-candida list such as tea, orange, wheat and milk (this is on the anti-candida list because of its milk-sugar content, but on its own it is often a cause of symptoms of cystitis) are causes of cystitis in their own right.

It is important to say here that I have never yet seen a person suffering from recurrent cystitis who did *not* have either candida or an individual food allergy. Because I do not confine my investigations to candida and food allergies, I find some of my patients also have a problem with the mercury in their dental fillings, a high body level of lead, aluminium, copper or cadmium, or are reacting adversely to some environmental agent such as North Sea Gas, petrol and diesel fumes, formalin, perfumes or house dust.

I look at all these and deal with them accordingly. While they may be playing a part in some people, they are seldom a major factor in chronic cystitis, although in the presence of a mercury problem candida albicans may be difficult to get rid of. As far as you are concerned, however, dealing with your candida and/or food allergies will rarely fail to help you.

When clinical ecologists find patients are allergic to certain foods, part of the treatment at some time involves a programme of desensitization. The methods used vary, but the principal is to make it possible for you to eat foods you are currently reacting to without them causing symptoms.

If you continue to eat foods of no nutritional value, such as sugar, white bread, tea, coffee or junk food, but under cover of desensitization, you will not have learned good eating habits. Part of the reason why you are now ill is because you have eaten the wrong foods in the past, some of which are now having a particularly harmful effect upon you, as well as creating nutritional deficiencies.

Although I gave a complete guide to candida diagnosis in Chapter 6, you will find a check list in the appendix that will help you decide if candida is possibly, probably or almost definitely involved.

If you decide to adopt the anti-candida diet, as I believe most women will, but also suspect certain other foods from the preference chart, combine the two. You will note that the Stone Age diet is not only an anti-candida diet, but goes even further. However, there are many foods that you need not avoid, if you decide to go on the anti-candida diet (when you will cut out such items as tea, coffee, orange and wheat) instead of adopting the Stone Age diet. Such foods are rice, corn (maize), soya, decaffeinated coffee, beef and pork.

The most difficult choice of all is whether to go the whole hog and try the five-day fast or not. Before starting, read my description of it again and, in particular, check whether it is suitable for you and what the pitfalls are. Done properly, it can be magic. Involve your husband or a close friend who knows you and will support you throughout. Write down what the problems are as you see them. Work out how long it will all take. I would advise you to set aside about six weeks to get through to the end. The first two weeks after actually commencing the fast are the most vital.

Check your diary ahead for important events. If you have a dinner in the near future, will it be possible for you to eat only those foods you have identified as being safe? If you are overweight now, will you have a dress or outfit that will fit you *when* you are so much slimmer? If you have always wanted to go on a diet to lose a lot of weight, as well as cease your suffering from recurrent cystitis, perhaps the five-day fast is just what you need. If you are *underweight*, however, please do NOT do the five-day fast without a clinical ecologist helping you.

Whichever method of altering your diet you choose, plan it properly and look ahead. Make sure you know what you can and cannot eat. Make lists of what you are allowed, and decide what you will eat at which meal. You will also need to plan what you are going to give your family if you have one. Remember, you must not handle flour if you decide to avoid wheat. If you are accustomed to baking, give it a miss for now.

Make sure you have adequate stocks of foods you *are* allowed to eat, and that you know where to get them from. Plan ahead to make sure that foods you want in a few days time are available. Above all let the family know. Post lists of what you are *not* allowed, and ask them to keep an eye on you.

If possible ban from the house foods you are not allowed. With a husband and children this may not be so easy. If you are on your own, put into a box all the foods in your cupboard you will be avoiding, and take them round to a friend. If they are not available at home it is easier to resist them.

Make sure you have some Epsom Salts and sodium bicarbonate available. Potassium bicarbonate is fine, but it is not so easy to obtain in small amounts. It can be swapped dose-for-dose with Epsom Salts. Buy a water filter or obtain adequate supplies of bottled water, and make sure you will be able to obtain more when you need it.

Remember, if for some unfortunate reason you have not cured your cystitis by one or more of the means I have described, your general health should definitely have benefited. If you are sensible you will adopt many of the ideas for good, and stay on a much healthier diet, so from this point of view the exercise will have been worthwhile. Because there *always is* an explanation for your cystitis, you have merely not found it. You may now *need* to find someone to help you, so one or more of the self-help groups may be worth contacting for the nearest practitioner.

PHASE 3

A word of caution is needed here. If you go onto a very restricted diet, please do NOT stay on it for long. It is not my intention that you should become a dietary hermit. I merely want you to find out the cause of your cystitis, and improve your general state of health. A very limited diet for too long can itself lead to nutritional deficiencies and produce a vicious circle. The more deficient you become the more your immune system will be compromised and the more allergies you will develop.

Get back onto as wide and nutritious a diet as possible, continuing to avoid those foods you find precipitate an attack of cystitis. If they are foods normally considered valuable such as orange, wheat or milk (although I personally have serious doubts about cow's milk and believe that almost everyone will be better avoiding it), let them back into your diet after three to six months of avoidance on a once or twice a week basis *at the most*, and see what happens. If you start developing cystitis again, you can always cut them out.

Provided you do not need to avoid too many foods, you should not run into any nutritional difficulties. In my opinion, if you are not a vegetarian or vegan, you are perfectly safe avoiding tea, coffee, citrus fruits, wheat, rye, oats, barley, junk foods and all cow's milk products such as milk, butter, yoghurt and cheese. The problem is, can *you* tolerate these limitations? Vegans and vegetarians are often very knowledgable about diets, but many do not realize they run the risk of zinc and vitamin B12 deficiencies in particular. If they were to have to avoid wheat, rye, oats and barley (the gluten-containing grains) their diet would be thrown into confusion.

If at any stage you want to get back onto a particular food but find on doing so your cystitis comes back, you will need to be desensitized to it. I have no intention of going into this process in this book as it is not something you can do for yourself. Unfortunately you will have to find someone to help you.

Finally, having made up your mind, stick to it. Read the book again while you are doing whatever you have chosen, and the best of luck!

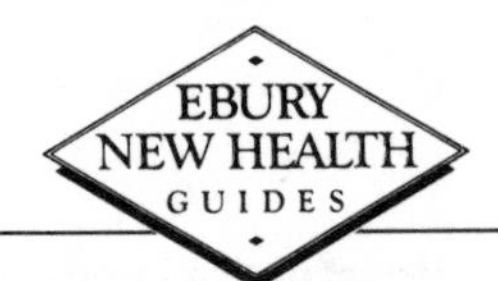

APPENDIX

IS CANDIDA THE CAUSE OF YOUR CYSTITIS?

Below is a check list to determine whether candida is *possibly*, *probably* or *almost definitely* a major cause of your cystitis.

	yes	no
1 Have you had a lot of antibiotics, either recently or in the past?	☐	☐
2 Do you suffer from premenstrual tension, or painful or irregular periods?	☐	☐
Do you have or have you suffered from endometriosis?	☐	☐
Do you have cysts in your breasts?	☐	☐
3 Have you been on the contraceptive pill for more than one year, or are you on it now?	☐	☐
Have you had hormone replacement therapy for more than one year, or are you on it now?	☐	☐
4 Have you ever had corticosteroid drugs, such as prednisolone, dexemethasone, betamethasone, ACTH injections?	☐	☐
Have you ever had three months or more of inhaled steroids such as Beconase for rhinitis, or Becotide or Bextasol for asthma?	☐	☐
5 Have you had three or more pregnancies?	☐	☐
6 Do you suffer from persistent thrush?	☐	☐
7 Do you suffer from symptoms such as mental confusion, mental fatigue, loss of concentration, forgetfulness, depression or mood swings?	☐	☐

8 Do you suffer from periodic or regular skin problems such as chronic urticaria (hives), psoriasis or fungal infections such as athletes' foot, or a rash between your buttocks or in your groin? ☐ ☐

9 Do you suffer from abdominal symptoms such as pain, bloating, constipation, diarrhoea, wind or indigestion? ☐ ☐

10 Do you suffer from cystitis, or a soreness or itching in the vaginal area, vaginitis or loss of interest in sex? ☐ ☐

11 If you are a man, do you suffer from prostatism? ☐ ☐

12 Do you suffer from headaches, muscle and joint pains or incoordination? ☐ ☐

13 Do you crave sugar, sugary foods such as chocolate or sweets, or yeast foods such as cheese, bread, alcohol or vinegar? ☐ ☐

14 Do you feel generally unwell with a number of vague minor symptoms that no-one can explain? ☐ ☐

15 Do you feel unwell in damp or mouldy conditions such as cellars or caves, or in damp weather? ☐ ☐

Do you feel unwell when gardening especially in winter? ☐ ☐

16 Do you have multiple allergies, and react to chemicals in the environment such as petrol and diesel fumes, North Sea Gas or perfume? ☐ ☐

Questions 1 – 4

- If you answer 'yes' to 1 question, candida is *possibly* a cause of your cystitis
- If you answer 'yes' to 2 questions, candida is *probably* a cause of your cystitis
- If you answer 'yes' to 3 questions, candida is *almost definitely* a cause of your cystitis

Questions 5 – 16

- If you answer 'yes' to 3 questions, candida is *possibly* a cause of your cystitis
- If you answer 'yes' to 6 questions, candida is *probably* a cause of your cystitis
- If you answer 'yes' to 9 questions, candida is *almost definitely* a cause of your cystitis

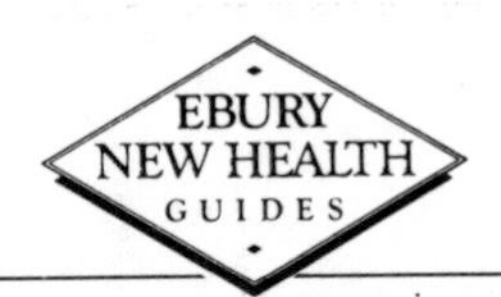

INDEX

Page numbers in *italic* refer to the illustrations